Understanding Interprofessional Working in Health and Social Care

Theory and Practice

Edited by

Katherine C Pollard, Judith Thomas and Margaret Miers

palgrave
macmillan

First published 2010 by
PALGRAVE MACMILLAN

Palgrave Macmillan in the UK is an imprint of Macmillan Publishers Limited, registered in England, company number 785998, of Houndmills, Basingstoke, Hampshire RG21 6XS.

Palgrave Macmillan in the US is a division of St Martin's Press LLC, 175 Fifth Avenue, New York, NY 10010.

Palgrave Macmillan is the global academic imprint of the above companies and has companies and representatives throughout the world.

Palgrave® and Macmillan® are registered trademarks in the United States, the United Kingdom, Europe and other countries

ISBN 978-0-230-21679-2

This book is printed on paper suitable for recycling and made from fully managed and sustained forest sources. Logging, pulping and manufacturing processes are expected to conform to the environmental regulations of the country of origin.

A catalogue record for this book is available from the British Library.

10 9 8 7 6 5 4 3 2
19 18 17 16 15 14 13 12 11 10

Printed and bound in Great Britain by
CPI Antony Rowe, Chippenham and Eastbourne

I dedicate this book to my father, J.J. Thomas MPS,
who was a model for interprofessional working,
and my mother Joan, a lifelong learner and teacher.

Judith

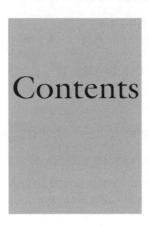

Contents

Acknowledgements

The editors wish to express their gratitude to all those individuals who con-tributed to the material presented in Part 1. We are particularly indebted to Professor Jonathon Benger, Margaret Boushel, Daphne Branchflower, Dr Toity Deave, Dr Judith Jones, Lois Pryce, Enid Smith and Dr Sebastian Yuen.

Notes on Contributors

Yusuf Ahmad is Principal Lecturer in Social Policy and Joint Programme Director of the MSc Leadership and Organisation in Public Services at the University of the West of England Bristol. His research interests include leadership, organization and delivery of public services. He leads a multidisciplinary team developing a leadership programme for senior adult social care managers.

Paul Godin is Senior Lecturer in Sociology at City University, London. His research activities have involved investigation of the work of community psychiatric nurses and forensic mental health care, from the perspectives of both professionals and service users. Paul's publications include *Risk and Nursing Practice* in Palgrave's *Sociology and Nursing Practice Series* (2006).

Tim Harle is an associate consultant at Bristol Business School, University of the West of England Bristol, where he directs the groundbreaking short course, Leading through Complexity. He was a senior executive in a FTSE-100 company and has contributed to three books, including *John Adair: Fundamentals of Leadership* (Palgrave, 2007). Tim studied at Cambridge University and INSEAD.

Celia Keeping is a social worker in a Community Mental Health Team in North Somerset and is also a Senior Lecturer at the University of the West of England Bristol. As a social worker her specialist area of practice is psychoanalytic psychotherapy. She is interested in the biographical roots of professional identity and the impact on interprofessional working.

Margaret Miers is Professor of Nursing and Social Science, Faculty of Health and Life Sciences, University of the West of England Bristol. She is series editor of Palgrave's *Sociology and Nursing Practice Series* and author of *Gender Issues and Nursing Practice* in the same series (2000).

Billie Oliver is Associate Head of School of Health and Social Care, University of the West of England Bristol. Her specialist subject areas include community development, youth work, informal education and group work. As Faculty strategic lead on Integrated Children's Services, Billie is currently researching the capacity of integrated children's practice settings to support learning for development in new roles.

Margaret Page is a Senior Lecturer in Organisation Studies at the Bristol Business School, University of the West of England Bristol, teaching on various postgraduate and undergraduate programmes. Her current research explores leadership and interpretation of requirements to promote gender equality within public services. In her work, Margaret develops arts-based inquiry methodologies for leadership, learning and change in organizations.

Katherine C Pollard is a Research Fellow in the Faculty of Health and Life Sciences at the University of the West of England Bristol. Her research interests include professional and workforce issues in health and social care, service delivery, interprofessional learning and working, and service user and carer experience. Katherine has a professional background in midwifery.

Derek Sellman is Principal Lecturer in the School of Health and Social Care at the University of the West of England Bristol. Derek's interests include education for professional practice, health care ethics, and philosophy of nursing. Derek is currently editor of the journal *Nursing Philosophy*.

Judith Thomas is a Principal Lecturer in Social Work in the Faculty of Health and Life Sciences at the University of the West of England Bristol. She is joint editor of Palgrave's *Interprofessional Working in Health and Social Care* and an author of the e-learning resource *Interprofessional and Interagency Collaboration* available at www.scie.org.uk.

Introduction: Background and Overview of the Book

Katherine C Pollard

Interprofessional working in health and social care is a topic of interest and importance for all of us in our various roles as students, workers, service users and/or carers. As Barrett *et al.* (2005:1) say:

> The nature of health and social care is such that, for many, the quality of the service received is dependent upon how effectively different professionals work together.

In *Interprofessional Working in Health and Social Care: Professional Perspectives – An Introductory Text* (2005), Gillian Barrett, Derek Sellman and Judith Thomas compiled accounts of the nature of interprofessional working from a comprehensive range of professionals. The aim of the book was to provide readers with an overview of the variety of ways in which interprofessional working in health and social care can be undertaken, together with an appreciation of relevant factors applying to particular professions and/or occupations. This text is a companion volume to that work. By drawing on a wide range of theory, it aims to help readers to develop their understanding of the complex process that is interprofessional working, including consideration of factors other than particular professional perspectives *per se*. Although the two books stand alone, together they offer readers the opportunity to engage with relevant issues in both breadth and depth.

Background to interprofessional working

Interprofessional working in health and social care is a concept which has received interest and attention for a considerable period of time in Westernized societies. In the USA, collaborative practice between health professionals has been advocated since the late 1940s (Baldwin 2007). In 1978, a global need was recognized in this regard when the Alma-Ata declaration on primary care recommended that health and social care professionals and agencies work together with local communities to improve service delivery, in order to promote public health and wellbeing (WHO 1978). Over the intervening thirty years, this standpoint has been embraced across the world, and a range of initiatives and policy directives have been implemented at both national and local levels, in order to promote better co-ordination, co-operation and communication between various service providers, service personnel and service users (see for example Miller 1997, Lazarus et al. 1998, Akhavain et al.1999, Romanow 2002, Meads and Ashcroft 2005a, Baldwin 2007, Bélanger and Rodriguez 2008, Bradley et al. 2008, Willumsen 2008). Initiatives have been diverse, and changes have not only occurred within existing services, but also across the public and private sectors, with innovative economic and structural models for health and social care delivery being trialled in various countries (Meads and Ashcroft 2005a). A common feature of innovative service delivery involves cross-boundary working, in which a range of workers take on the performance of tasks and duties previously associated only with a particular health or social care profession (see for example Lumsden 2005). In this way, these tasks and duties have been redefined as being based on competence rather than profession, in that occupation alone does not determine who conducts them (Cameron and Masterson 2003). Such cross-boundary working relies on effective interprofessional collaboration for its success.

Consideration of initiatives implemented across the world makes it apparent that interprofessional working can take many different forms. However, a common feature of interprofessional working is that it requires active engagement between various representatives of different professions and occupations in order to be successful.

Over the years there has been much debate and discussion about what the term 'interprofessional' actually means. As various standpoints have been well-rehearsed elsewhere, they will not be presented here again. Interested readers are referred to Pollard et al. (2005) for wider discussion of this issue. Throughout this book, a basic meaning of 'interprofessional working' or 'collaborative practice' is understood as

> the process whereby members of different professions and/or agencies work together to provide integrated health and/or social care for the benefit of service users.
>
> (Pollard et al. 2005:10)

This definition does not, however, allow for active contribution on the part of service users/patients/clients to processes of decision-making concerning care delivery. It should be noted that current thinking about interprofessional working demands that the service user voice should also be heard in interprofessional forums and situations (Thomas 2005).

In the UK, government policy since the late 1980s has both advocated and insisted upon effective collaboration between all those involved in health and social care – agencies, service providers, professionals, support workers and service users, in varying combinations (see for example Great Britain 1989, 2004, Welsh Assembly Government 2005, Department of Health 2008a, 2008b, Department of Health, Social Services and Public Safety 2009, National Health Service Scotland 2009). High-profile problematic cases, such as those concerning Christopher Clunis (Department of Health 1994), the Bristol Royal Infirmary (Kennedy 2001), Victoria Climbié (Laming 2003), Alisha Allen (Carvel 2008) and Baby P (Laming 2009), have also driven the interprofessional agenda. These cases have illustrated how serious consequences can ensue when services are not sufficiently well co-ordinated, and when systemic factors adversely affect satisfactory care delivery. Service response has at times taken the form of organizational restructuring, and many policy documents outline planned services whose success appears to be entirely dependent upon effective interprofessional working. For example, Department of Health (2006:8) states that

> There will be more support for people with long-term needs. People with long-term conditions will be supported to manage their conditions themselves with the right help from health and social care services. ... To support a more integrated approach we will develop Personal Health and Social Care Plans and integrated social and health care records. To help people receive a more joined-up service, we will be establishing joint health and social care teams to support people with ongoing conditions who have the most complex needs.

As is obvious from the above, these targets can only be met if health and social care workers are working well together. However, the situation on the ground is far from clear-cut, with accounts of both effective and difficult interprofessional working still being reported (see, for example, Glasby et al. 2008, Hansson et al. 2008, Miller et al. 2008, Pullon 2008).

Over the last decade, there have been numerous research studies focusing on interprofessional working, investigating what it entails and what renders it (in)effective (see for example Miller 1997, Cook et al. 2001, Booth and Hewison 2002, Hudson 2002, Lane 2005, Carmel 2006, Pollard et al. 2008, Miller et al. 2008, Pullon 2008). Nevertheless, there have been fewer attempts to theorize this area so that underlying principles, issues and factors can be understood in a manner which enables the development of knowledge and transferable skills among service organizations and the human beings who interact within them. This need has been recognized, however, and the body of theoretical work concerning interprofessional issues is now growing (see for example D'Amour *et al.* 2005, Meads and Ashcroft 2005b, Couturier *et al.* 2008). This book aims to contribute to this body of work, concerned as it is with *understanding* interprofessional working in health and social care.

Overview of the book

In order to help increase such understanding, the editors have drawn together both a variety of accounts of interprofessional working and a variety of theoretical perspectives from which to consider relevant issues. It should be remembered that the implementation of interprofessional working within health and social care is not isolated from wider social influences. Factors which affect society as a whole also affect the way that individuals working within the health and social care services operate in relation to their own roles, to colleagues from other disciplines and to service users. The book therefore considers interprofessional working in relation to theoretical perspectives developed in the context of studying broader issues such as values and ethics, processes of identity formation, interpersonal interaction and communication, changing professional boundaries, the process of medicalization, and the constitution and operation both of organizations and of wider society.

The book is divided into two main parts. Part I, 'Different places, different voices', contains a range of material comprising individuals' thoughts and responses concerning their own experiences in relation to interprofessional working (Chapters 1 to 5). These accounts reflect how diverse professions, occupational groups, care settings and care groups can be. The service user voice is also included in Part I.

Part II, 'Analysing the issues', focuses on theoretical understanding of factors arising within interprofessional working (Chapters 6 to 12). In each chapter, interprofessional working in health and social care is discussed in relation to a specific theoretical area. Space constraints have inevitably resulted in omissions, but the editors have aimed to present a range of theories in this section, including both those which address particular professional issues, and those which apply to wider societal perspectives.

The book ends with a concluding chapter, in which the author identifies implications for services, service providers and service users arising from the issues raised in Part I and the analyses provided in Part II. The further development of interprofessional working in health and social care is discussed in this context.

Throughout the book, readers are offered reflective activities in order to assist their engagement with the issues in question. Reflective practice is an accepted component of professional education: it provides not only an opportunity for serious questioning and critical thinking, but also the means whereby learners may become aware of how their own personality and/or emotions influence their perceptions and actions (Boud and Walker 1998). The editors hope that readers will use these activities to further their understanding of relevant issues.

Making the most of the book

The material in Part I provides the reader with a variety of examples and opinions expressed by different individuals operating in the health and social care arena. As a collection of portrayals of interprofessional working, these accounts are by no means exhaustive or representative of collaborative practice. However, they are authentic accounts of real situations and events, given by real individuals either receiving, organizing or delivering health or social care in the UK. The editors suggest that readers take the opportunity to read these 'voices' attentively, in order to get a sense of some of the different contexts in which interprofessional working can occur, and of the issues which can arise. Reflective activities are provided at the end of each chapter in Part I, in order to help readers think about influencing factors and possible consequences associated with the examples of interprofessional working presented in these individual accounts.

In Part II, chapter authors have drawn on the range of material presented in Part I to illustrate their discussion. Theory in each chapter is explored and illuminated by reference to individual 'voices' in Part I, in order to provide an authentic context for specific points of interest. The reader will note that in some places, different chapter authors in Part II have used the same material from Part I to illustrate quite different themes, and have even interpreted material differently. The editors feel that this demonstrates how diverse perceptions of events and issues can be among individuals considering collaborative practice in health and social care.

It should be noted that any phenomenon can be understood and discussed from a variety of vantage points. For example, there is ongoing debate about whether interpersonal or professional factors have more influence within interprofessional interaction. The likelihood is that both are extremely important, but that one may take precedence in particular circumstances. Readers are invited to consider the different theoretical perspectives presented in Part II, and with reference to the material in Part I, to make their own decisions about which theories are most useful in aiding understanding of the process of interprofessional working in health and social care. Exercises are presented throughout each chapter in Part II, in order to encourage readers to consider issues from their own vantage point, and to help them to enhance their understanding of this important aspect of health and social care practice.

References

Akhavain P, Amaral D, Murphy M, Uehlinger K, Cardone M (1999) Collaborative practice: a nursing perspective of the psychiatric interdisciplinary treatment team. *Holistic Nursing Practice* 13(2):1–11.

Baldwin DeWC Jr (2007) Some historical notes on interdisciplinary and interprofessional education and practice in health care in the USA. *Journal of Interprofessional Care* 21(1) Supplement 1:23–37.

Barrett G, Sellman D, Thomas J (2005) Introduction. In: Barrett G, Sellman D, Thomas J (eds)

Interprofessional Working in Health and Social Care: Professional Perspectives – An Introductory Text. Basingstoke:Palgrave Macmillan,1–4.

Bélanger A., Rodriguez C (2008) More than the sum of its parts? A qualitative research synthesis on multi-disciplinary primary care teams. *Journal of Interprofessional Care* 22(6):587–97.

Booth J, Hewison A. (2002) Role overlap between occupational therapy and physiotherapy during in-patient stroke rehabilitation: an exploratory study. *Journal of Interprofessional Care* 16(1):31–40.

Boud D, Walker D (1998) Promoting reflection in professional courses: the challenge of context. *Studies in Higher Education* 23(2):191–206.

Bradley F, Elvey R, Ashcroft DM, Hassell K, Kendall J, Sibbald B, Noyce P (2008) The challenge of integrating community pharmacists into the primary health care team: a case study of local pharmaceutical services (LPS) pilots and interprofessional collaboration. *Journal of Interprofessional Care* 22(4):387–98.

Cameron A., Masterson A. (2003) Reconfiguring the clinical workforce. In: Davies C (ed) *The Future Health Workforce*. Basingstoke:Palgrave Macmillan, 68–86.

Carmel S (2006) Boundaries obscured and boundaries reinforced: incorporation as a strategy of occupational enhancement for intensive care. *Sociology of Health and Illness* 28(2):154–77.

Carvel J (2008) Death of shaken baby raises parallels with Baby P case. *Guardian* December 6 www.guardian.co.uk/society/2008/dec/06/shaken-baby-durham-social-workers (Accessed 7.12.08).

Cook G, Gerrish K, Clarke C (2001) Decision-making in teams: issues arising from two UK evaluations. *Journal of Interprofessional Care* 15(2):141–51.

Couturier Y, Gagnon D, Carrier S, Etheridge F (2008) The interdisciplinary condition of work in relational professions of the health and social care field: a theoretical standpoint. *Journal of Interprofessional Care* 22(4):341–51.

D'Amour D, Ferrada-Videla M, Rodriguez LSM, Beaulieu M-D (2005) The conceptual basis for interprofessional collaboration: core concepts and theoretical frameworks. *Journal of Interprofessional Care* 19(Supplement 1):116–31.

DH (1994) *The Report of the Inquiry into the Care and Treatment of Christopher Clunis*. London: The Stationery Office.

DH (2006) *Our health, our care, our say: a new direction for community services*. London:DH.

DH (2008a) *High Quality Care for All: NHS Next Stage Review Final Report*. Chair, Lord Darzi. CM 7432. London:The Stationery Office.

DH (2008b) *Putting People First - working to make it happen: adult social care workforce strategy - interim statement*. www.dh.gov.uk/en/Publicationsandstatistics/Publications/Publications PolicyAndGuidance/DH_085642 (Accessed 29.04.2009).

DHSSPS (2009) *Families Matter: Supporting Families in Northern Ireland. Regional Family and Parenting Strategy*. www.dhsspsni.gov.uk/families_matter_strategy.pdf (Accessed 08.04.2009).

Glasby J, Martin G, Regen E (2008) Older people and the relationship between hospital services and intermediate care: results from a national evaluation. *Journal of Interprofessional Care* 22(6):639–49.

Great Britain (1989) *Children Act*. London:The Stationery Office.

Great Britain (2004) *Carers (Equal Opportunities) Act*. London:The Stationery Office.

Hansson A., Friberg F, Segesten K, Gedda B, Mattsson B (2008) Two sides of the coin: General Practitioners' experience of working in multidisciplinary teams. *Journal of Interprofessional Care* 22(1):5–16.

Hudson B (2002) Interprofessionality in health and social care: the Achilles' heel of partnership? *Journal of Interprofessional Care* 16(1):7–17.

Kennedy I (2001) *Learning from Bristol: The Report of the Public Inquiry into Children's Heart Surgery at the Bristol Royal Infirmary 1984–1995.* London:The Stationery Office.

Laming, Lord (2003) *Inquiry into the Death of Victoria Climbié.* London:The Stationery Office.

Laming, Lord (2009) *The Protection of Children in England: A Progress Report.* Norwich:The Stationery Office.

Lane K (2005) Still suffering from the 'silo' effect: lingering cultural barriers to collaborative care. *Canadian Journal of Midwifery Research and Practice* 4(1):8–25.

Lazarus J, Meservey PM, Joubert R, Lawrence G, Ngobeni F, September V (1998) The South African Community Partnerships: towards a model for interdisciplinary health personnel education. *Journal of Interprofessional Care* 12(3):279–88.

Lumsden H (2005) Midwives' experience of examination of the newborn as an additional aspect of their role: a qualitative study. *MIDIRS Midwifery Digest* 15(4):450–7.

Meads G, Ashcroft J (2005a) Policy into practice: the case for. In: Meads G, Ashcroft J, with Barr H, Scott R, Wild A, *The Case for Interprofessional Collaboration in Health and Social Care.* Oxford:Blackwell, 36–57.

Meads G, Ashcroft J (2005b) Policy into practice. Collaboration. In: Meads G, Ashcroft J, with Barr H, Scott R, Wild A, *The Case for Interprofessional Collaboration in Health and Social Care.* Oxford:Blackwell,15–35.

Miller K, Reeves S, Zwarenstein M, Beales JD, Kenaszchuk C, Conn LG (2008) Nursing emotion work and interprofessional collaboration in general internal medicine wards: a qualitative study. *Journal of Advanced Nursing* 64(4):332–43.

Miller S (1997) Midwives' and physicians' experiences in collaborative practice: a qualitative study...Models of collaborative practice: preparing for maternity care in the 21st century. *Women's Health Issues* 7(5):301–8.

NHS Scotland (2009) *A Force for Improvement: Workforce Response to Better Health, Better Publication.* www.scotland.gov.uk/Publications (Accessed 09.04.2009).

Pollard K, Rickaby C, Miers M (2008) *Evaluating student learning in an interprofessional curriculum: the relevance of pre-qualifying interprofessional education for future professional practice.* HEA Health Science and Practice Subject Centre with UWE, Bristol. www.health. heacademy.ac.uk/projects/miniprojects/completeproj.htm (Accessed 7.12.08).

Pollard K, Sellman D, Senior B (2005) The need for interprofessional working. In: Barrett G, Sellman D, Thomas J (eds) *Interprofessional Working in Health and Social Care: Professional Perspectives – An Introductory Text.* Basingstoke:Palgrave Macmillan, 7–17.

Pullon S (2008) 'Competence, respect and trust: key features of successful interprofessional nurse–doctor relationships'. *Journal of Interprofessional Care* 22(2):133–47.

Romanow R (2002) *Building on Values: The Future of Health Care in Canada.* Ottawa: Commission on the Future of Health Care in Canada. www.hc-sc.gc.ca/english/pdf/ romanow/pdfs/HCC_Final_Report.pdf (Accessed 13.10.2006).

Thomas J (2005) Issues for the future. In: Barrett G, Sellman D, Thomas J (eds) *Interprofessional Working in Health and Social Care: Professional Perspectives – An Introductory Text.* Basingstoke:Palgrave Macmillan,187–99.

Welsh Assembly Government (2005) *Designed for Life: Creating world class Health and Social Care for Wales in the 21st Century.* www.wales.gov.uk/subihealth/index.htm (Accessed 09.04.2009).

WHO (1978) *Primary health care. Report of the International Conference on Primary Health Care, Alma-Ata, USSR, 6–12 September 1978. (Health for All Series No. 1).* Geneva: World Health Organization.

Willumsen E (2008) Interprofessional collaboration: a matter of differentiation and integration? Theoretical reflections based in the context of Norwegian childcare. *Journal of Interprofessional Care* 22(4):352–63.

PART I

Different Places, Different Voices

Introduction
Judith Thomas and Katherine C Pollard

In the following five chapters we have gathered a range of voices from individuals either working in or using different English health and social care organizations. All material presented has either been specially commissioned, drawn with acknowledgement from previously published research, or comprises data/findings from studies where, before participants consented to take part, they were informed that their contributions would be published in a variety of media. Some chapters draw heavily on a research programme concerning interprofessional education undertaken at the University of the West of England, Bristol. All the research referenced in Part I received ethical approval from university and/or NHS research ethics committees.

This section offers a selection of individual 'voices', in order to provide readers with a sense of issues, situations and events which can be associated with interprofessional working in health and social care. Owing to space constraints, the selection is not exhaustive, and some readers may be disappointed that their own profession or occupation is not represented. Indeed, there has been no attempt to collect contributions from a 'representative' sample of health or social care professionals. As this section is not designed to provide 'evidence' for interprofessional working, but rather to provide illustrations of individuals' experience of collaborative practice, the editors have chosen to include contributions from practice areas and individuals for various reasons. Contributions from individuals involved in community care, children's health care, emergency care and the interface between primary and acute care settings have been included because these practice areas have undergone considerable restructuring in recent years as a result of government policy (Great Britain 2003, DH, DfES 2004, DH 2006, Alberti 2007). Maternity and mental health services are represented because they are areas in which the concept and extent of service user involvement in care delivery have been particularly highlighted and debated over the years (DH 1998, Page and Hutton 2000, Hope 2002, DH, DfES 2004). Service user involvement is obviously of key importance in the current context of care delivery, as is the involvement of the voluntary sector (increasingly referred to as the third sector). In each area addressed, the editors have solicited material from individuals who between them inhabit many relevant professional roles.

Professional role is, however, only one factor influencing interprofessional collaboration in health and social care. Wider social factors also play a part, notably gender, ethnicity, culture and religion. While both men and women have contributed to Part I, the editors could not ensure representation based on other social factors, often because of demographic constraints affecting study populations. We acknowledge this as an omission, but consider that the material presented still offers a broad range of perspectives for readers to explore.

The voices

Chapter 1, 'Care in the community', considers three contrasting scenarios in community care. First we hear from an occupational therapist and a community nurse, both working in recently integrated community teams. They consider the team development and issues relating to role development and overlap. The impact of different management structures and systems, including those relating to finance, are also discussed.

The second scenario illustrates the work of a health visitor and a general practitioner (GP) who highlight how changes in policy and practice impact on their roles, and the adjustments they are making to accommodate the changing landscape of health and social care services. The GP's reflections on the interface between primary and secondary care lead on to the third scenario in which a social worker and an adult nurse discuss communication challenges relating to discharge from hospital.

Chapter 2, 'Care in acute settings', considers the challenges of interprofessional teamworking in the context of emergency care, acute care settings for children and the care for older people in hospital, including discharge back into the community. Differences between short- and long-term teams, problems with rotation, and the influence of traditional practices and hierarchies are considered. The interviewees refer to the necessity for independent professional judgement, autonomy and delegation, while also needing mature teamworking skills to ensure safety through effective written and verbal communication, challenge and debate. The chapter discusses the particular pressures and challenges created by legislation and policies, such as those relating to timing of discharge from hospital and waiting times. The interviewees question whether these changes influence working practices, necessitating greater degrees of integration. The narrative accounts also illustrate how professionals' perceptions of their own role, team and capacity for change compare with colleagues they perceive as having more ingrained working practices.

In Chapter 3, 'Service users, carers and the voluntary sector', we hear the voices of service users, carers and voluntary (third)-sector workers. The chapter starts with the reflections of a service user who considers how recent developments in policy and practice affect her. A carer articulates her concerns with the way she and her mother were treated by different professionals. A range of different individuals reflect on their experiences of working more collaboratively with people who need services and their carers. Differences between user involvement and user-led services and what these mean in the context of collaborative working are highlighted.

The community development worker interviewed starts by commenting on the lack of understanding of what is meant by 'the voluntary sector' and offers clarification. Interviewees in this chapter have been involved with government programmes such as Sure Start that aims to deliver the best start in life for every child by bringing together early education, childcare, health and family support. Others have worked with charities including Home-Start, through which parents support other parents and families experiencing the effects of postnatal illness, disability, bereavement, the illness of a parent or child, or social isolation.

In Chapter 4, 'Maternity and infant care', midwives, medical practitioners and mothers consider how the personality, character and experience of professionals contribute to their ability to work with others. Differences between settings offering similar services are explored in terms of atmosphere, the varying degrees of formality and levels of intervention in pregnancy, labour and postnatal care. The way in which differences of opinion are resolved and the extent to which parents are involved in this process are considered. Drivers for changes in working practices, including those resulting from staff shortages and different levels of expertise in particular techniques are considered. Interesting issues emerge from the interviewees relating to power and authority, connecting particularly to the boundaries and overlaps in the role of midwives and junior doctors.

Chapter 5, 'Mental health care', focuses on mental health care services. The chapter considers the widespread call for interprofessional working within mental health care policy and professional literature. It starts with the views of mental health nursing students who consider the factors they perceive as influencing interprofessional collaboration. These are followed by a social worker's reflections on collaboration with a consultant psychiatrist, which reveal the importance of utilizing a range of professional skills and demonstrate how professional training develops specific 'ways of seeing' that bring different insights to individual difficulties. The importance of the 'whole picture' is particularly well illustrated here. An interview with another social worker highlights an example of communication failure, highlighting the distress professionals can feel when collaboration fails. This complex case involved a range of organizations and raises issues about the consequences of failure for future inter-agency relationships. In contrast, a qualified mental health nurse describes positive interprofessional working in a setting providing day therapy for people with eating disorders. The chapter concludes with the perspectives of managers, nurses, psychologists, psychiatrists, service users and an occupational therapist who consider risk, blame and the reality of collaborative working in a forensic mental health care unit.

Making the most of Part I

Part I aims to provide readers with a range of individual accounts which can act as a resource to illuminate issues, situations and attitudes which may influence or arise from interprofessional working. We invite readers to complete the reflective activities given at the end of each chapter, and hope that they will stimulate deeper thought and wider ideas about influencing factors and possible consequences associated with interprofessional working in health and social care.

References

Alberti G (2007) *Emergency care ten years on: reforming emergency care.* www.dh.gov.uk/en/ Publicationsandstatistics/Publications/PublicationsPolicyAndGuidance/DH_074239 (Accessed 10.04.2009).

DH (1998) *Modernising mental health services: safe, sound and supportive.* London:Department of Health.

DH (2006) *Our health, our care, our say: a new direction for community services.* London:Department of Health.

DH, DfES (2004) *National service framework for children, young people and maternity services.* London:Department of Health.

Great Britain (2003) *Community Care (Delayed Discharges etc.) Act.* London:The Stationery Office.

Hope T (2002) Evidence-based patient choice and psychiatry. *Evidence Based Mental Health* 5:100–1.

Page LA, Hutton E (2000) Introduction: setting the scene. In: Page LA (ed) *The New Midwifery: Science and Sensitivity in Practice.* Edinburgh:Churchill Livingstone, 1–4.

1

Care in the Community

Material collated by
Judith Thomas and Katherine C Pollard

In this chapter, we present voices of practitioners involved with community care. Interviews were conducted with a health visitor and a recently retired GP specifically for this book. Other material has been drawn from two research studies undertaken to evaluate interprofessional education for pre-qualifying health and social care students (Pollard et al. 2007, 2008).

Service scenario 1

The first two excerpts demonstrate practitioners' views of new community teams, in which services for health and social care are jointly managed and delivered.

Occupational therapist (1): integrated community team for people with learning difficulties

'The multidisciplinary team [MDT] here works extremely well together. I've been here an awfully long time so I've seen quite a few of the changes . . .the support for the professionals here comes from the [MDT] team . . . it's a very flat structure within the team...most people are on face-to-face terms, we're on the same sort of playing field so that makes it a lot easier . . . We have a lot of joint working . . . so I work very closely with the physios, group therapy, community nursing . . . we have a lot of blurred barriers . . . so that makes quite a big difference I think when you're working very closely face-to-face . . .

I don't think anybody in the team feels really threatened by it [role overlap] . . . we have team meetings where we discuss clients . . . we decide who's going to do what and how it's going to be done . . . we have a way of negotiating it, but we do have quite clear overlaps. I deal with physiotherapy quite a lot . . . and [the physiotherapist] does a lot of postural management and seating . . . we overlap quite a lot on who provides walking aids and wheelchairs and specialist seating and we do a lot of joint visits . . . sometimes it's just a really hard case and we both go just to bump heads together and cry over it and say we don't know what to do . . . She sits on the specialist seating sub-group . . . it's quite new for a physio to sit on that, so if I apply for seating, specialist seating, and it's over and above the normal amount then it goes through a special seating panel and she's started to sit on that . . .

We mix people's skills and we do that with community nursing as well, we've got a community nurse here we work quite closely with and a psychiatrist . . . there's been a necessity to work with people – whereas in a department you can fall back on your department colleagues . . . here you haven't got that so you're a lot more forced to do it . . .

We've got some very strong personalities within the team . . . the social workers are quite new to the medical side of things, they tend to be quieter in the meetings because they've only just joined us . . . the clinical meetings have actually changed to service users' meetings and lost the name of the clinical meetings to make [the social workers] feel more comfortable with it and I think they still really don't know the purpose of the meeting and what they should be discussing in the meeting and what they shouldn't, so they're holding back a bit . . . we've got staff that have been here a long time and a bit more experienced that then do take the lead on the meetings but I think . . . that people are actually now thinking . . . how can you involve other people and help them feel more comfortable? . . . We have some professionals, they only join the meeting occasionally . . . when they actually arrive at the meeting it's dedicated to them . . .

The meetings are really to almost document sometimes people's concerns and issues . . . most of the work is done outside [the meeting]. We're all based in the same place and that helps considerably. So all the offices are upstairs . . . the offices are broken up into different – not into same professions. When we first moved in people had psychology rooms and the OT room and it was disastrous, and it was a conscious thing on the teams when people left and we re-jigged the whole thing, the social workers came in recently so everybody moved offices so that instead of the social workers moving into established offices where people knew each other well, everybody is new. There's a social worker in each office . . . we have mixed professions in each office, so that there's not this sort of ghetto . . . everybody leaves the door open and so we have quite a lot of conversation which is really helpful . . . the teamworking is more important than their professional role or you know, status within it. . . . We'll link with anybody if it's in the best interests of the client and I think that's what the team focuses on, if it's in the best interests of the client then they will liaise with anybody and facilitate that working . . .

We're a pooled service, so we're financially pooled, budgets, and our management structure has changed . . . originally . . . we were managed by profession, everybody had a professional hierarchical structure and we had a head of profession and then it went to the Chief Executive . . . so it was a very simple structure. Now . . . the district manager . . . he's my line manager, and then I have a clinical manager . . . who's an occupational therapist, so that's quite a big change . . . we've had a slow move away from the professional system towards this sort of local district manager position. The thing that happened with the integration and what people were very concerned about was that the council have a different style of management to the NHS and the NHS trusts were very worried because they saw that the council style is quite dictatorial from top-to-bottom, tight structure and they were fearful of decisions being taken away from them and being organized at a management service level, whereas here the decisions have always been made by the team, or the team members held the budgets for us and organized the way things happened. And of course the budgets were then removed . . . so that the budgets now are held by the district manager.

. . . what is probably happening is the big management attitude change, is that the team are . . . almost moulding their manager . . . it's a steep learning curve for both sides. [The practice manager] can be thinking he's a manager and he needs to manage . . . whereas we don't actually see it in that way, we see him as more of a consultative person . . . so it's difficult . . . I think over time the team members have shown their work and their knowledge and their experience and that they can contribute to decision-making and that it's probably best if [the management] let us know if there is a problem within the service and then we can consult on it and offer some advice . . . I think initially people were quite defensive but now they're sort of trying to do more positive action, to try and mould things and change things round . . . and we've had some decisions which he has reacted quite badly to, and I've actually stood up and said, "Oh no, we're not going to have this" . . . the trouble is that before, we had very clear information, and I think now under this different style of management we don't get all the information . . .

Usually the team tends to take a team response to it, so out of that incident [replacing a medical secretary with an ordinary secretary] there was a team letter that went to our service managers . . . asking for a response to get answers why they took the decision the way they did. And the response was, well it's in the agreement with the PCT that we do that, and so then people said, "Well, we don't know anything about this," . . . so it's now gone back to our PCT . . . it still needs to be a medical secretary . . . we then also feed into our professions because each one of us on the team has a service lead who sits on the service managers' meetings . . . I think they'll be a bit more careful in the way they do things in the future because it's caused a bit of ill feeling . . . the managers we've got now are social services managers so they're not totally aware . . . he's doing the job descriptions, he's now on the physio job descriptions, and he's only just now saying, "Well really, I didn't realize that physios did this and this and this and this" . . . they're very unaware of what each professional does because they've come from managing social workers...he's managed one profession, and we're not one profession we're lots of different professions, with all different standards and all different rates of pay and working hours and conditions . . . [they're] on a steep slope really, so they can't make decisions for all the professionals . . . '

Community nurse: intermediate home care team

'The documentation is all . . . one folder within the patient's home whilst they're under our care and one folder in our offices and we have a daily handover meeting . . . to ensure that we are talking to the other members of the multidisciplinary team. Oh, we also have support workers who work with us . . . who are actually physio-assistant and OT-assistant trained. So as well as doing the basic personal care . . . they also do follow-up with the therapists . . . follow-up exercises, follow-up programmes that the therapists set . . . as do the nurses, in fact. If there's a therapy programme that needs doing on a day that a nurse visit is planned . . . rather than sending in two or three different people then the nurse will actually follow the therapy programme as well . . .

We wouldn't set a programme but we would follow instructions from another therapist. So if somebody has had a hip replacement and the physiotherapist set them specific exercises . . . we would just follow those instructions and assist in doing them. And if there was a . . . side effect of pain then, obviously, we would be able to assess and provide the intervention necessary for that. So there is this . . . sort of . . . overlap . . . having a knowledge of what a person is having to be put through and what impact it's going to have on them from the nursing side of things. And we can just involve each other in whatever aspects of care we are providing for that patient . . .

From the nursing point of view it's the assessment, I would say. And again it works from two different aspects in that you've got the rehab [rehabilitation] of . . . for instance . . . a stroke or hip replacement which are fairly formatted . . . the emergency interventions could be a lot more variable and you can have to attend . . . sometimes on a daily basis if somebody needs assessing on that daily basis . . . to make sure that any other intervention from other professionals is being provided appropriately . . . it might be because they need their stamina building up so we would then refer on to the physiotherapist. It might be that they've suffered a bereavement . . . it's something that maybe a CPN [Community Psychiatric Nurse] could help with . . . you know . . . bereavement counselling or something like that.

. . . [non-nursing professionals] might come across somebody who has been incontinent and would have to deal with it. They might come across somebody who is in extreme pain and call a nurse in . . . there have been occasions when wounds have oozed . . . and all our physios carry basic gloves and maybe a basic tape and gauze so that at least they can patch something up and then call for somebody else . . . they wouldn't necessarily assess and put the specific dressing on.

. . . we've just moved offices and prior to the move . . . the professionals were separated from the support workers and it was quite difficult . . . the last two months since we have moved have been wildly different from the prior ten months and really, now, I would put [our interprofessional working] at 8/9 our of 10. It really is spot-on. The support workers feel much more supported and that they are being listened to . . .

I think in hospital you don't get a true picture of what a physio and an occupational therapist really can do in the community . . . and what an occupational therapist can do to keep somebody [in their own home] . . . it can be very specific to that person's needs.'

Service scenario 2

Two professionals central to providing community health care are the health visitor and the GP. The former's remit is promoting health and preventing ill health, in the broadest sense, through identifying and addressing health needs. Health visitors are employed by NHS Primary Care Trusts (PCTs). Some are geographically based, and some are attached to GP surgeries. They work in health-care settings and in service users' homes. Their client group usually comprises pre-school children and their families; they have a statutory obligation to see all babies between 10 and 14 days old.

In the following excerpts, a health visitor and a GP speak about working with other professionals and services, including role overlap resulting from the development of other practitioners' roles..

Health visitor

'The health visitor is the team leader, and there may be nursery nurses . . . health visitor assistants or community nurses who are registered nurses, but don't have a community qualification . . . playworkers . . . [all employed by the PCT]. The people that you work with and/or refer to will be midwives, school nurses, GPs. If you've got some elderly on the caseload, or some unwell mother, it might be the district nurse, but that might be through the GP anyway, depending on your relationship. Social services are a very prominent one . . . referring to CAMHS [Child and Adolescent Mental Health Service], audiology, those sort of medical or allied health professionals . . . '

. . .

'What is your role is in relation to the other people in the team?'

' . . . if we talk about a new baby . . . if it's a new birth, and there's an older child, say maybe two years old, and there's problems there, mother's not really knowing about play, what the best things are to do . . . I'll go back to the clinic, I'll tell the mother, "Would it be OK with you if the playworker comes along, just to talk through that?" . . . I would discuss the family with the playworker and say, "Look, you go in and see what the mother's levels of play are, what her knowledge is, etcetera, and maybe do four visits to get her started or to see how it goes." She wouldn't have responsibility for that family . . . You'd never expect them [playworkers] to take responsibility for giving advice outside the remit that they are competent to do, because most of them work within specific competencies. Really, the health visitor won't necessarily have all the contacts with the family, but will have the overall remit for that family . . . [the health visitor is] the core, the main person, really. Because you can be held accountable by courts, social services, whoever.'

'*How do you find working with social services?*'

'It's often been problematic because of their workload. You will refer someone in, and you won't hear anything from it . . . sometimes they seem a bit heavy-handed; and that's usually when you don't know the social worker very well. I've found that when I've got to know the social workers well, or on a professional basis really, you get some sort of working relationship and occasionally do joint visits together, which can be beneficial. But it's always, if you mention social workers to health visitors they all go, "Oh God, they never respond" . . . In many areas, local authorities, there'll be a referral team, so you refer to the referral team, and it's up to them to decide what to do with it; and if you think it's a priority then you've got to make a really big case for it to be actually acted on . . .

I don't think they mean to be obstructive. They just . . . their priorities aren't necessarily the same as ours . . . I think it depends on how much contact you've had with them. Say, for example, where I was working before I came down here, on a very deprived estate, what I highlighted as a need . . . would be very different from what health visitors in the south of the city would . . . And social services know where you're referring from, and may know vaguely the family situation, or that area situation, and may think, "Oh, not a problem; the health visitor says it is, but . . . ". If it comes from the GP as well, maybe from someone else, then it's a priority – well, it doesn't work quite like that, but it's always been problematic, and I think it always will be, just because our demands, our priorities are different.'

'*What about the relationship with the GP?*'

'That's always been problematic – no, there are some GPs and health visitors who work very well together. GPs might not work very closely with their health visitors but when they are...well, not threatened really . . . but when the PCT says, "We're going to place all our health visitors in a community clinic, they're going to be geographically-based, etcetera," GPs fight it . . . I have never worked particularly closely with GPs . . . I've only liaised with them when I've felt that they should know about something. But, bar one or two instances, I've never had a GP ringing me up saying "I'm concerned about . . . ", even although I've worked mainly in very deprived areas with very high needs . . . in [one area], where they were single-handed most of the time, I was fighting against a lot of the advice they gave . . . I was never invited to any of their meetings – I didn't necessarily want to go, but they didn't seem to include geographically based people. When I was living in [another area], there was a GP who started doing a surgery in a clinic where I was . . . I always had very good relationships with them . . . so it's quite varied.

Relatively recently . . . they [GPs] realized that if we did the immunizations then they would get extra money . . . Sorry, I'm being very cynical there, but it does seem to have gone along with, where money goes, health visitors become a little bit more popular.'

Skill mix has always been seen as a threat, because you have these lower-paid people coming in, and a health visitor post goes, that's how it's been perceived. The idea is that they complement each other, and they're a stronger team . . . the playworker, the community nurse, the health visitor assistants, etcetera. Whereas before there was just a health visitor, with maybe a health visitor assistant. It was brought in, and it wasn't made explicit, and it was seen as a watering-down, rather than a boosting-up . . .

You've got this split between education and health, with education saying, "Yes, these people [health visitors] are really important", through to the other departments saying, "Well, actually they're not." They're not being recognized, or the money's not getting through. There's been a lot of change and a lot of insecurity, so health visitors are . . . desperately trying to hold on to what they know they can do, and not wanting others to do assessments for them, etcetera, keeping that responsibility. And that's quite difficult when you've got a multiprofessional team, and you're meant to be working together.'

GP

'The people under one roof were the nurses, doctors and admin. There were regular weekly meetings...we shared problems a lot on daily basis . . . because of our varying expertise of up to twenty years we looked at a lot of scenarios and it was a useful forum to just come and troubleshoot. . . .

What we learnt was really quite patchy; sometimes doctors were not very clear about how they should involve other agencies . . . now it is very clear-cut, one is expected to follow the guidelines... There is more onus on GPs to be aware what is expected and not just do what they think, because at the end of the day they have to be accountable . . . the days when you could make up what you think and play it as you want are no longer, and you really do have to follow the guidelines.
. . .

A lot of children-at-risk case conference requests come in weekly . . . Those sort of meetings take a lot of time, a huge pressure . . . You had to choose ones where you have a lot to say and ones where you had been very involved. .. Having said that if you don't go you are expected to fill in the form. The quality of those forms was quite variable and some doctors don't take them as seriously as they might. . . .

District nurses were the most interwoven with our practice, they see our patients all the time. They have a lot to say; we used to have weekly meeting for about one and a half hours, but some doctors didn't think it was a good use of time. They come and bring in samples for pathology most days; we communicate through a message book. They have been a stable team, therefore we get to know them well – any slight problems, anything they are concerned about, they tend to catch us when they come into the surgery. It is very different with midwives, they tend just to contact us when they have a problem. Nowadays midwives are much more independent practitioners than they used to be, linking much less with GPs. This is a point of contention as the GP's role is much less than it used to be . . . I don't think the changeover went very smoothly because we went from a situation where our practice was very hot on obstetrics – we had a licence to work at the local hospital and do our own deliveries; two of us were competent to do low-risk forceps delivery at the hospital as well as home delivery. We had a local antenatal clinic and were very involved but then felt elbowed out as midwives got more organized and better trained. I think they felt they could do what we were doing . . . so there was some animosity...The change has taken away some of our expertise as if you don't use your skills, particularly in obstetrics, you get rusty. . . . they [patients] can go through whole of a pregnancy and the next time the doctor sees them they have got a baby . . . [doctors] feel a bit miffed . . .

I don't see any tensions with our own [practice] nurses [who] have got more and more skilled. There is a big overlap between what we do and they can do, particularly when dealing with minor illness. We run a telephone triage system...the doctor or the nurse phones the person back, in our system the doctor phoned back. Nurses run triage, so if someone has a bad throat or a bad ear, we let nurses look at that. Even a bad chest if they are trained to deal with it. We see that nurses have been pushing to have more of a clinical role and are moving away from minor nursing tasks that they are giving to health care assistants, and nurses are coming to overlap more with doctors. Some doctors are a bit worried about this, I have heard doctors comment, "Where is this going to end; are these nurses trying to be doctors?" We have to appreciate they are training up and there is a big overlap . . .

We set up our system with doctors doing it [phoning back] because of personnel who we had at the time...nurses work much more from protocols than doctors and we know from out-of-hours' experience that nurses aren't disposed as much as doctors to be able to conclude something on the telephone . . . it may be about risk taking, once [a doctor] is experienced. The surgery were rather loath to move to nurse triage as we would have more people to see . . . a doctor will deal with up to 80 per cent on the phone, whereas there is a different ratio for a nurse . . .

[Patients have] expectations around who you will see and who will provide treatment . . . a lot in terms of building expertise and expectations. One example of that is cervical smear tests. You used to only get that through a doctor, now nurses do that and an internal examination is part of that. People phone in for a test and expect the doctor to do something and are quite surprised when they are told the nurse will do that . . .

There could be more interaction with social workers and I've always had good relationships with them but I do feel there is a bit of us and them . . . Some doctors are afraid to get involved with social issues, don't see it as their job . . . doctors are worried about confidentiality, there are huge issues about,

"What can I tell the social worker; I know there is a risk here . . . but what ball will it start rolling?" These were the sort of issues that people would bring to coffee-time discussions. What can I tell social services, what action would I be entering into? There is no room for an off-the-record discussion . . .

Medical problems relating to social issues with older people . . . who may be being abused come up regularly. District nurses tend to flag up these sort of issues. It was an issue for people in their own homes and in residential care. Sorts of things like, is the patient falling or being pushed in their own home, why are the patient's wounds not healing? Who is tampering with it, is some one else doing it? Patients who get lacerations, how did they get them when they can't move?

. . . [It is important] knowing at what point you have suspicion . . . worthy of involving another agency. You need to do that only when there really is an issue, and then being very clear what the issue is . . .

The forms from social services for child protection and adults at risk are not good for GPs, they are designed for lots of different agencies. They need to be more specific with sections just earmarked for doctors, so it is clear what part of the form GPs fill in . . . '

'*Were there any issues about admissions and discharges?*'

'Huge problems and around the waiting-list problem. We spend a lot of time trying to be the patients' advocate. There was a lot of messing around with certain types of patient. Failed paperwork, people being sent out too early and bouncing back in too readily. Failures getting in, failures getting out. Patients not knowing what was happening. . . . Admissions cancelled, notes lost and the doctor's letter getting lost. A lot of people who go in and don't really understand what has happened, don't know what it was they had done, that's a communication issue. Sometimes they would come in into the surgery weeks later with ECG [electrocardiograph] leads still on their chests, patients thinking it was part of treatment to have these plastic things stuck to them . . .

The way things have moved, there is a tranche of their [doctors'] work that can be done by other people, and one of the most important things is, for doctors to survive they have to give away some of their work... doctors have to be trained that they are part of an interdisciplinary team, while they have a lot of good skills they happen to be different. One of the things they might be able to do is draw things together in a way that perhaps others in a team can't particularly, if there is a big medical issue involved; but if you are going to survive in medical teams you have to value every member of that team for what they have to offer. I think that's where training has to be going and the sooner medical students are introduced to that idea the better.'

Service scenario 3

As mentioned by the GP (above), the interface between primary and acute care is a key area in care co-ordination. In the final excerpts, two hospital-based practitioners speak about difficulties encountered when service users were being discharged from hospital.

Social worker(1): hospital, community care discharge assessments

Social worker(1) feels that interprofessional collaboration impacts on both the patient and their relatives as they need to know what help they are getting and what is going to happen to them. She gave an example of how poor interprofessional collaboration had impacted on a patient who was due to be moved and said, 'Things like this happen every day.' The patient had MRSA [methicillin-resistant staphylococcus aureus][1] and C-DIF [clostridium difficile][2] and therefore needed barrier nursing. Social worker(1) did the specialist assessment and the discharge team arranged the transport. When the ambulance arrived it refused to take the patient because he had MRSA and C-DIF and they had another patient on board. The patient was elderly and was very confused by what was going on – he thought he was leaving that day. Social worker(1) said, 'How much can you take as a social worker?' The discharge team are qualified nurses and social worker(1) felt that it should have been their responsibility to make sure that transport was aware of the patient's condition. She said, 'Sometimes you feel as although you have to treat everyone as although they're stupid.'

Adult nurse(1): acute medical ward, respiratory specialism

'We recently had somebody we had to get home and it's a palliative issue and they needed to have home oxygen but not all the time . . . it was going to be a future need, obviously, as their condition deteriorated . . . but in the initial stages it wasn't necessary . . . but anxiety meant that they felt they needed oxygen and they were worried about being able to do the stairs and things. And just by working together with the lung cancer nurse specialist . . . and the respiratory care nurses, the physiotherapist and the OT [occupational therapist], just to get somebody to learn that they could do the stairs by stopping halfway up . . . they had deep-breathing techniques for anxiety . . . the lung cancer nurse specialist to say, "I will be in touch the day after you've got home, when you've settled in. I've ordered the oxygen and it will be in on Monday . . . "; by ringing the district nurse to say they're going to come out on Monday when the oxygen arrives . . . just to get that person home on a Friday rather than sit in hospital till the Monday – that it happened involved a lot of people and experience in knowing who can help . . . that's the essential . . . that maybe you can make somebody's stay shorter or improve the package when they go home . . . it makes a heck of a difference.'

Summary

These accounts of working in health and social care in community settings illustrate changing patterns of care delivery and the challenges professionals face when working together, particularly when working closely with colleagues to bridge 'divides' that have arisen through ways of organizing and financing care. For example OT(1) describes working in an integrated health and social care team, organized to focus on the needs of people with learning disabilities. Those working in the integrated team experience changes to management structures, changes in place of work, changes in individual roles. You may find it helpful to make a list of the changes OT(1) identifies.

REFLECTIVE ACTIVITY

Reflect on why such changes might be important for collaborative working. Does the community nurse working in the intermediate home care team identify any ways of working collaboratively that are similar to those described by OT(1)? Drawing on your own experience, can you think of other practices that would support good interprofessional working at a time of change?

In contrast to Service scenario 1, the interviews with the health visitor and the GP suggest that bridging the health and social care divide is not easy. Similarly the examples in Service scenario 3 illustrate the challenges involved in ensuring service users can have a positive experience of moving from hospital to home-based care. What issues do these professionals identify as creating difficulties for clients and professionals? What strategies would you suggest to resolve such issues and to remove barriers to effective collaboration?

You may find it helpful to return to these questions and answers after you have read each chapter in Part II.

Notes

1 An infectious disease, resistant to antibiotics.
2 An infectious disease associated with diarrhoea and abdominal pain, to which older people are particularly vulnerable.

References

Pollard K, Rickaby C, Miers M (2008) *Evaluating student learning in an interprofessional curriculum: the relevance of pre-qualifying interprofessional education for future professional practice.* HEA Health Science and Practice Subject Centre with UWE, Bristol. www.health.heacademy.ac.uk/projects/miniprojects/completeproj.htm (Accessed 7.12.08).

Pollard K, Rickaby C, Ventura S, Ross K, Taylor P, Evans D, Harrison J (2007) *Transference to Practice (TOP): a study of collaborative learning and working in placement settings. The student voice.* Bristol: University of the West of England. http://hsc.uwe.ac.uk/net/research/Default.aspx?pageid=29 (Accessed 7.12.08).

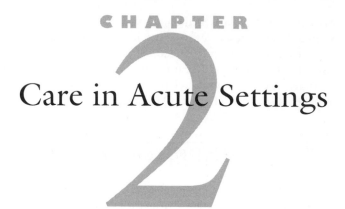

CHAPTER

2

Care in Acute Settings

Material collated by
Margaret Miers and Katherine C Pollard

In this chapter we present excerpts from staff working in acute settings. The emergency care consultant and the senior registrar working in paediatrics were interviewed specifically for this chapter. All other interviews were conducted as part of a longitudinal evaluation of a pre-qualifying curriculum. This evaluation followed students through to qualified practice (Pollard *et al.* 2007, 2008).

Service scenario I

An adult nurse and a consultant report on their experiences of working in accident and emergency departments and pre-hospital admission emergency care settings. Both describe emergency care as characterized by effective teamwork and report on the development of new roles and practices designed to provide satisfactory care within time pressures.

Adult nurse(2)

'We've got our own set of doctors that are always placed in A&E [accident and emergency] so obviously we work alongside them . . . patients will come in off an ambulance, well paramedics as well . . . initially the nurses will see them first unless they are really, really unstable, they'll do sort of triage [assessing people in terms of medical need] . . . Like if it was chest pain, obviously we'd do observations, ECG [electrocardiogram] all that sort of thing, bloods, and then once we've kind of finished, we will then introduce them to the doctor and sort of say you know, "This is his ECG, these are his observations, we've sent these bloods and ordered him a chest X-ray", but then the doctor will come in and sort of do their thing, so we work quite closely with them really. . . .

When [interprofessional working] is working well, it's really successful, especially with community liaison becoming a bigger part of it now and the physios are quite happy to come down and assess . . . originally it was just A&E and if we needed [patients] to be assessed and we needed them to be seen by community liaison it would have to be a medical admission . . . so you were then getting people that probably could have gone home but would be admitted because we didn't have that relationship with those professions that could come and see them, but now that we do, we can ring them up and . . . they'll come and assess the mobility and say, "Yeah, they're perfectly fine with a frame, we're happy for them to go home", and the community liaison nurse will come in and say, "Yes, that's fine, we need somebody to come in, we can arrange that . . ." and then they can go home that day. So it does work really well.'

Emergency care consultant

'The role of the consultant in an emergency department is to oversee the management of all the patients by all the staff . . . you are not necessarily always physically present, but you are still responsible for what goes on. I often tell the juniors that one of the key skills about being a consultant is not about delivering good clinical care when you are there, it is about delivering good clinical care when you are not there. It is about setting up systems and processes that facilitate high-quality management . . . what you have to do is delegate. You have to trust people to be doing the right thing . . . this relies on a number of professionals working together and it particularly relies on the relationship between doctors and nurses because we rely on the nursing staff to work with the medical staff to flag up issues and problems so one of the key features – it is a bit like the crew resource management issues in aviation – is to create a safe environment. So we empower the staff – "Are you sure about that? Is that the right thing to do?" – to ask questions. And therefore the student nurse can ask the consultant, in an open atmosphere, "Why are you doing that?" . . .

If you look at the way that we work the roles are quite interchangeable so there are things where it is not clear whose responsibility it is. For example . . . if the medical staff are busy, the nursing staff take blood. If the nursing staff are busy, the medical staff take blood. It doesn't really matter, does it? What's important is that somebody does it and it fits into the overall workload of the department . . . patients come into the department and we share our documentation. It is a single record and the nursing staff write in it and the medical staff write in it. It reduces duplication . . . '

'Your processes and systems would allow, under some conditions, some nurses to order the X-rays?'

'Yes, whenever you encounter a barrier, the thing is what is getting in the way of this patient's care right now? A lot of this is being facilitated by the time pressures, in terms of having a four-hour target, that means you have to look very hard at your processes . . . one of the enablers is to ensure that the people who might need to request that investigation are able to do so . . .

. . . we've done a lot of work . . . to build up the role of physiotherapy in the department, particularly in terms of seeing people autonomously from the queue. So an experienced, properly trained physiotherapist will see a patient with a knee injury, for example, will see, assess and treat those patients and discharge them without recourse to any other practitioner. And of course one of the problems we came across really early on was X-rays. A lot of people need X-rays . . . wherever possible we'd encourage the practitioners themselves to develop their own [training] programmes but they often need the medical rubber stamp . . . '

'So . . . what becomes the problem is legitimacy with other departments?'

'Yes . . . there'll always be anxiety about allowing another profession to request an X-ray . . . although we have had a lot of success with this, even some of my colleagues have been persistently reluctant – "Ooh, I don't know about this . . . ", depending on their mindset. . . . [there are] anxieties around the issues, particularly around whether it impacts on training . . . particularly if you have a lot of nurse practitioners, as we have . . . who are seeing minor injuries then it means that your medical staff don't get expertise in minor injuries . . . we are not entirely clear how we are training people for the future . . . '

'You were emphasizing safety and making sure everyone has a say . . . '

'Yes, well, teams make for safer patient care. When you have multiple people involved in a single process it gives you multiple checks and balances in a system and it stops people doing something very abnormal. One person, thinking in an illogical way, not thinking very clearly in a situation, if they have a lot of power they can make a lot of mistakes . . . Major medical errors occur often because of a combination of circumstances which allow one person to do something catastrophic, so where you have got multiple team members you can achieve much higher levels of safety in patient care . . . '

'Could I just ask you a little more about the skills, the interpersonal skills, of working well together?'

'It requires a certain type of individuals to work well in teams, obviously. I think emergency care works well with this because . . . emergency care is a low level in terms of prestige as a medical speciality and it is a relatively new speciality. There's not too much of an ingrained hierarchy so the expectation of those being trained in the speciality is not that they are going to be called "Sir" and wear a white coat and [be] followed around by a long trail of juniors. So the role modelling for the trainee is all about kind of integration, teamworking, etcetera, etcetera, and we work very hard with the trainees to look at such things as communication skills, interpersonal working . . . People who are poor communicators or people who aren't very good at getting what they want done in a way that is polite and effective get into all sorts of trouble.

. . . It helps if you are not too egotistical and if you are relatively relaxed about things in terms of kind of not too anxious about the way things are done. There are ways of getting things done and it is just a question of finding those routes that work. Standing around and shouting at people doesn't work very well. So communication becomes a key issue. It is about team ethos and atmosphere. We have to be quite careful sometimes with the juniors. It is difficult for the junior doctors, increasingly difficult for the junior doctors because they are very junior and they don't really know a lot. The nursing staff know a lot more than they do. It is very good for the juniors to work in that environment but they find it quite different from a ward, where the traditional hierarchy still seems to run true . . . they do have to develop their skills and make decisions so the negotiation skills in terms of getting what you want in a way that is acceptable...it really hones people . . .

. . . we're doing a lot of pre-hospital care recently . . . at the scene, that might be quite complicated and quite uncontrolled, you have a number of ambulance personnel, for example, and the actual lines of who is in charge are quite clear. The ambulance personnel are in charge of the medical response but the medical response brings a certain degree of expertise. The police and the fire service on the scene all just expect the doctor to be in charge of the medical response, but the ambulance service might subscribe to a different view. Getting what you think needs to be done for the patient and getting it done in a way that doesn't cause a complete kind of breakdown at the scene is a huge skill . . . you are with people you have never met before and have to form teams in a very short space of time and that is a real development of the same skill concepts. How do you make teams work? How do you get things done effectively in a way that allows everyone to contribute, using their skills in a way that doesn't undermine the whole process of care? Because the determination to keep control can be undermining to the quality of care.'

'*And in those circumstances, it is the emergency services that are in control?*'

'Well, it is very complicated. The police are in overall control of the scene and the fire service are in control of the bit right next to the patient. But in terms of the medical response . . . the doctor at the pre-hospital scene is under the control of the ambulance service . . . But you get the situation where the patient is critically ill and needs medical intervention, and it might be that the ambulance personnel on the scene have a different view, and therefore making that tick is quite challenging, and delivering high-quality care and feeling good about it can be a big challenge because you have to form a team on the spot.'

'*So . . . it is essential to have those teamworking and diplomacy skills.*'

'Yes, because it is not about, "I'm the person in charge, I'm the top of the hierarchy therefore I decide what you do and you do what you're told." It doesn't work. It is not appropriate and neither does it deliver good care because of the risk of error incurred. People aren't empowered to speak up, people aren't being used in a functioning team. So that kind of model is outdated . . . but the problem is to change that model to one of team forming, communication, teamworking, which I think gets much better results in the long run, people just find very threatening. They feel that it undermines their power or their self esteem . . . that it will undermine status and position. I think it is frankly rubbish because people don't give you respect on the basis of how loud you can shout or what your title is or what you are wearing. Respect is something that is earned through a completely different process . . . People fall back on this hierarchical cushion because it makes them feel comfortable . . .

. . . Dare I say it, I suspect that with increasing numbers of female doctors we will see increasingly better teamwork. We are a bit stuck in the "male doctors, female nurses", underlying gender issues, there's a kind of hierarchy that seems to be perpetuated. But with increase in medical graduates being women . . . I expect that means we'll see better teamworking. There'll be less egotistical approaches . . . For myself, I feel comfortable in my role and secure in what I am doing so it doesn't matter. What I am interested in is actually the team and the communication and the delivery of care.'

Service scenario 2

A senior children's nurse and a senior registrar working in paediatrics report on their experiences of working in acute settings for children. The nurse works in a paediatric unit comprising two specialities. Nurses work across both specialities which are at different 'ends' of the ward. The senior registrar works on a general paediatrics ward in a large acute hospital but he reflects on his experiences of working in a range of settings. Excerpts from the interview with the children's nurse have been previously published (Pollard 2009).

Children's nurse

'From my opinion interprofessional working works, from a children's nurse point of view . . . Obviously junior nurses are different to senior nurses and as a senior nurse, I have got a lot of experience so I can make a lot of decisions and then go to the relevant person . . . I think the interprofessional relationship we've got is good. From the respect of junior doctors knowing who the senior nurses are, and obviously seeking them out to ask their opinion rather than just dictating, "This is what I want you to do" . . . they don't often recognize the difference between a senior nurse and a junior nurse . . . we all look the same. . . . So in that respect, the interprofessional nursing relationship, I think is very difficult for junior nurses and I think that it can knock their self-esteem and confidence because doctors have asked them to do something . . . then they have to seek help from senior members of the team. . . .

When we merged before we came to the new unit . . . the general feeling was that this isn't going to work . . . the two specialities don't mix. There are only two commonalities about these specialities . . . they both have acute . . . . critical care aspects to them . . . the A end always think they are busier than the B end and the B end always think they are busier than the A end. . . . The B end is about post-surgical care, wound management, pain and then discharge and rehabilitation. The A side is ongoing, it's long-term. The priorities are different. The multidisciplinary team is different . . .

. . . With the A scenario you have key nurses, hopefully, you have the pain management team, the play specialist team, the occupational therapist team, the physiotherapist team, and then you've got clinical neurophysiologist coming in, the speech therapist coming in and the swallow team coming in. . . . and then you have the schoolteachers, so you have about nine individuals that are linked to that one child who the nurse has to pull together. The B end . . . obviously the consultants both sides, but . . . some consultants on the B side get very over-involved and try to dictate who is involved in the multidisciplinary team, and you've got play specialist, OT, physio . . . When the child is going home on the A side, the clinical neurophysiologist stays on board, sometimes the physio . . . and then the school team. But what's lacking from both sides is that there is no A outreach person and there is no B outreach person.

. . . the multidisciplinary team for A – they are around for a long time. The OT . . . , the physio . . . the dietician is around for a long time, . . . Whereas, on the B side the OT comes and goes and then does a follow-up. The dietician comes and goes because the child generally improves really quickly . . . So the multidisciplinary team is short-acting . . . '

' . . . *I did go to one of the A meetings and I was struck by the way the team worked together . . . there did seem to be space for people to actually put their opinions forward . . . '*

'There always has been.'

'When I spoke with the students, they said they found the B team meetings huge and terribly formal . . . '

'It is. B team is consultant-led completely, but I'd say A team is half and half, half nurse and half consultant, or half ward and consultant . . . The B team meeting . . . is very formal . . . nurses can have their say but it's intimidating, it's threatening . . . I wouldn't say either of them is easier to deal with . . . I find it equally frustrating really, because of the . . . lack of communication really, from the team members and on documentation. . . . It's very difficult. The A side, I think, have just started that we are allowed to write in the child's medical notes and as long as we sign it, date it, time it, etcetera, do all the legal aspects, and the doctors are quite happy as long as we don't do nurse writing which is like reams . . . "keeping it concise" is the phrase. . . . I think the discharge planning on the B side is appalling to say the least . . . I don't think enough thought is being taken by junior nurses . . . communication is the biggest problem . . . the A side is more cohesive definitely, there seems to be more planning and more thought, but saying that, the A team is made up of very, very, very long-term experienced nurses.

. . . The A doctors, because it's mostly one [medical] team . . . you've got a very regular team. Now the B end again, you've got B doctors and plastic doctors and you've got orthopaedic doctors. So you've got three specialities down that end and the doctors come in at various times and in various ways, and the . . . orthopaedic doctors, like general surgeons, do not communicate unless they have to with anybody. And they will walk straight to the trolley or they will walk to a bed without even asking a nurse to come with them. Or they will ask any nurse to go with them whether it is their patient or not. There is this egocentric thing going on with orthopaedic doctors . . . if they can get away with speaking to a senior nurse, they won't speak to a junior nurse or a student unless they have to, unless I say, "No, this is who you need to talk to, they are looking after your patient" . . . Very odd, and I've come from a different trust, different hospital and it's not any different . . . I only qualified in 1993 and the orthopaedic doctors there are exactly the same as the orthopaedic doctors down here . . .

And they don't always write in the notes . . . we have to have ESP [extra-sensory perception], or we have to go and bleep them and say, "Oh, you popped in and saw so-and-so and you never wrote in the notes, who did you communicate with?", and they will say, "Oh, well we didn't", and we will say, "Right, so you need to either come back and write in the notes or come and communicate with somebody regarding this because we have now got a mother coming in to the nurses' station asking what's going on; and do we know what's going on? No, because you haven't told us, so now I'm bother-ing you and bleeping your pager to tell me what's going on." Dreadful, dreadful communication. . . . It's historical, it's ritual . . . '

Senior registrar, paediatrics

'The closest we work with is nurses, and in general, I think we have quite a good relationship . . . I would imagine that most doctors work along a doctor agenda and everything revolves around them, they feel they're busy and impor-tant, so they will turn up on a ward round, they expect nurses to drop what they're doing to attend the ward round and support them, and give informa-tion. We communicate as we come on to the wards, we should communicate if we've got any admissions or people going home, should communicate on ward rounds – better departments will have joint meetings. I personally feel that if you want things to work well, you will have joint everything, so joint han-dovers. That's what they do in the children's hospital . . . the nurse co-ordina-tor and maybe an outreach nurse from intensive care will come to the doctor handover twice a day, so they will be able to give their input on what they're worried about, and the bed state and parents and children, and learning what the doctors' plans are for the day, and they would inform that. Here, and like many hospitals, they don't have nurses in the handover – so we would first meet them when we come to the ward round in the morning.'

'What makes doctor–nurse relationships good?'

'We have a functional working relationship, so we try to communicate. The better doctors, the more experienced doctors, will do as they're told – and so in that way it functions. Nurses know what they want and they often tell us what to do, and we do it. I guess if there was any kind of fear, communication problems, then they wouldn't be able to tell us what was needed. Often you get a feel on the ward of how things are and often you can feel, because conversations are quite relaxed, things are informal, that things are going reasonably well . . . I think there's quite a lot of frustrations often as well, I think nurses think doctors don't understand their needs and their problems, and I think that they're probably right . . . A recent example was, it's more convenient for me and the family for the patient to come to me on the ward and see me; and I believe all children should be at home, so I send everyone home almost. Whereas the nurses, if a child steps through the front door, they need to be admitted, that's just the way the system is. Therefore that entails them filling in papers, putting some stuff on the computer; and if I keep them there for ten minutes, they then also have to be discharged – now I can tell them, "This child is not going to stay", but they feel, because the way the processes work, that – so that frustrates them sometimes . . .

We do have . . . multidisciplinary teams, and examples would include paediatric oncology, . . . cystic fibrosis or respiratory, particularly in the community, and CAMHS [Child and Adolescent Mental Health Service] . . . The specialist nurses would be at the heart of it . . . In general, those teams will have regular meetings . . . and we discuss each patient that's on the books, actively on care in the hospital, or active problems in the community; and that'll be like an hour-long meeting, we'll go through them all and people put their different bit of information in. So that's where things work well.'

'Is there much overlap between roles of doctors and specialist nurses?'

'Everything's changing, because what the government's trying to do across health care, and I think probably across all professions now, is look at what job needs doing, and see who's best able to do that – and there are different benefits, but I guess one is going to be a cost saving. So doctors can be great at doing many things, but there's quite a lot of stuff that they do that anybody could do, so they're making a whole load of new roles now; so traditionally if someone is injured or did something to themselves, they'd come to hospital and a doctor would see them and patch them up; but now you have emergency-care practitioners who used to be ambulance drivers . . . who now assess the patient in the house, and if they just need some first aid or simple advice, they would advise them to stay there . . . that's good, really, I like change, and I think that it frees up doctors to do different things, so I'm all for everybody getting extra training and doing things differently; because it's more efficient for the patient.'

Service scenario 3

A consultant geriatrician and a social worker report on their experiences of interprofessional working in an acute setting for older people. Both focus on issues involving patient discharge and reflect on policy and management changes that affect their work.

Consultant geriatrician: acute medical ward for older people

'We all have our roles . . . and I know that my role there is to talk about the diagnosis and the prognosis and what my expectations are as an overview, and then the nurse's role is to reflect on the nursing needs of the patient, but they also of all the team have the closest relationship with the families so they are a more direct bridge for the families . . . And then the physio's role is really very much about physical issues, about transfers, and mobility and stairs and things, and the OT again has a role, and a social worker does, but I think we all know what we have to bring to the meeting about each patient, we know what everyone else would expect us to know . . . what is fortunate is that . . . the nurse manager and her team and I have worked together for four and a half years, so we know each other very well, and you know that's a sort of very easy relationship . . . but the physios and OTs rotate and they're often only there for about six months and then they move on . . . I think what's quite nice is that they enjoy coming to an MDM [multidisciplinary meeting] where they can actually contribute and be listened to because I think that some MDMs . . . dependent on who's running it, they kind of don't get so much opportunity to chip in, sort of thing, and so they rise to that . . .

Social Worker A, I think has probably been with us for about two or two and a half years . . . Social Worker B is very much newer to us . . . she's finding her feet. We've had a bit of a reputation for sort of seeing off social workers . . . it's just because I think we work very hard as a team to keep people moving through. I mean from the second someone arrives on the ward we're thinking, "What are the discharge issues going to be?" . . . If you've got a social worker who sort of drifts up once a week . . . and they sort of get round to talking to the family two weeks later, it drives us nuts because the rest of us are pushing it through on a daily basis, and so we have got a reputation for being hard on our social workers. And people like Social Worker A who work hard anyway and you know has similar views fits in like a dream . . . but some of the other social workers . . . one actually did suggest that she was being bullied by us which I don't think was true at all, but that's her perception of it. So I think people like Social Worker B come to us slightly nervous . . . but she's . . . very, very good . . .

. . . because [the physios and OTs] change every six months, . . . at the end of the day what I require from them is factual information . . . so I just ask them for the fact if they don't contribute spontaneously . . . we did have a structure about, up until about 18 months ago, where we had our own physio and our own OT for the ward full-time which was wonderful . . . the team-work then was even stronger because they were just around and they knew everyone . . . we really need much more involvement from OT and I think we feel frustrated that if we had a full-time OT on the ward we would actually be getting people through more quickly . . . We've had it fed back to the OT manager and he's aware of it, but he's got manpower problems.'

'If that's happening, do you expect more of the nurses to do more of OT kind of skills?'

'Well, they do. I mean, there is quite a lot of generic work anyway. If you can double the mobilization, you know our nurses actually . . . are all very experienced . . . and they know how to transfer and mobilize people . . . the problem with – the OT role is very specific. I mean our nurses do things like wash and dress assessment . . . but things like home assessments and home visits they really can't get involved with . . . it's outside their experience and capability so we are still very dependent on OTs for that . . . if you were trying to set up a care package, and you want assistance with washing and dressing, Home Care [service] do expect an OT to have made that assessment . . . '

Social worker(2): hospital, community discharge assessment

'Do you feel there are any difficulties around boundaries?'
'Yes, there is a little bit. We have the discharge liaison team . . . they facilitate discharges from hospital. They challenge you continuously – are they ready, why the delay? Is it your delay? because of the hospital Discharge Act,[1] section 5 . . . In a way our roles are blurred because they will try to work around us, they'll find a vacancy at a nursing home for a particular person still in hospital. But we know it is completely inappropriate but they might have gone ahead and told the family, and it is quite difficult to undo all that.'

Service scenario 4

The final extract is from an interview with a physiotherapist who works across a range of wards in a hospital but is not attached to one setting. Organizational factors, including office location, appeared to affect interprofessional communication.

Physiotherapist: rotational hospital post

'I'd say there's a lot of communication breakdown . . . I very much see the physiotherapist/occupational therapist/dietician/speech and language therapist as a team and the nurses as a separate team . . . I find that actually within the other allied health professions we communicate very closely and work very well together but then it will inevitably break down when you need to involve some nurses . . . the attitudes are completely different . . . as I say, other professions *expect* to get on with . . . dieticians, speech and language . . . that group . . . whereas I don't think the nurses quite have that same ethic . . .

It's so frustrating when things fall apart . . . and it really impacts the patient. You can write in the nursing Kardex for days about something before it actually happens and you will always hear other members of staff griping over that . . . they'll have arranged a discharge for a patient . . . and it will completely fall apart because somebody didn't make a phone call along the way . . . it's always a communication breakdown . . . someone else thinks someone else is doing it and yes, it really impacts on service delivery . . . yesterday I'd seen a patient on a ward with COPD [chronic obstructive pulmonary disease] and I'd handed over to the nurses that the patient *must* be walked on oxygen to the toilet. And I happened to be on the ward later . . . the patient's SATS [blood oxygen saturation levels] were just ridiculous . . . 71 per cent[2] . . . because they'd taken him *on air* to the bathroom, even although I'd told them in the morning . . . I'd handed over to one but then they hadn't handed it between them . . . and that's a massive impact on service delivery.'

Summary

This chapter began with accounts of working in emergency care settings. The view of Adult nurse(2) is that when interprofessional working is working well 'it is really successful'. The emergency care consultant suggests that time pressures hone team-working skills. He supports non-medical professionals in developing their skills to extend roles in order to ensure the workload of the department is managed effectively. The senior registrar, paediatrics, also supports 'doing things differently' for the benefit of the patient. Other accounts of acute care settings, however, suggest that medical leadership styles vary considerably, with implications for the nature of teamwork. A key theme in this chapter can be seen as the professional perceptions of senior doctors.

REFLECTIVE ACTIVITY

The accounts offer an opportunity to consider the role of the medical profession in contemporary health and social care teams. Drawing on your own experience as well as the voices in this and earlier chapters, note down your observations on the influence of medical practitioners on interprofessional working. In addition, consider the working practices of other professional groups involved in acute care (physiotherapists, occupational therapists, social workers and nurses are all referred to in this chapter) and identify behaviours that facilitate or inhibit successful teamworking.

Review your observations after you have read each chapter in Part II.

Notes

1 Great Britain (2003) *Community Care (Delayed Discharges etc.) Act*, London: HMSO.
2 SATS should normally be above 90 per cent.

References

Pollard K (2009) Student engagement in interprofessional working in practice placement settings. *Journal of Clinical Nursing* 18(20):2846–56 DOI: 10.1111/j.1365-2702.2008.02608.x.

Pollard K, Rickaby C, Miers M (2008) *Evaluating student learning in an interprofessional curriculum: the relevance of pre-qualifying interprofessional education for future professional practice.* HEA Health Science and Practice Subject Centre with UWE, Bristol. www.health.heacademy. ac.uk/projects/miniprojects/completeproj.htm (Accessed 7.12.08).

Pollard K, Rickaby C, Ventura S, Ross K, Taylor P, Evans D, Harrison J (2007) *Transference to Practice (TOP): A Study of Collaborative Learning and Working in Placement Settings. The Student Voice.* Bristol: University of the West of England. http://hsc.uwe.ac.uk/net/research/ Default.aspx?pageid=29 (Accessed 7.12.08).

3

Service Users, Carers and the Voluntary Sector

Material collated by
Judith Thomas and Katherine C Pollard

In this chapter, we present views and experiences of care delivery from the perspectives of service users, carers, voluntary (third)-sector workers and other professionals concerning service-user and voluntary-sector organization involvement in service delivery. All the material was commissioned specifically for this chapter.

Service users and carers

Service user(1) is a wheelchair-user, and requires assistance with most physical activities

Service user(1) is in receipt of direct payment. This means that she does not access commissioned services, but receives money directly from Adult Community Care (ACC – social services) so that she can buy in the care that she wishes to receive. She has two full-time personal assistants, whom she employs. They follow a rolling rota, working three days at a time.

Service users are allocated to the direct payment system as a result of needs assessment. The assessment covers the following:

- What can you do for yourself?

- What care/services do you think you need?

- When do you think you need this care/service?

The assessment is conducted by a social worker, who usually comes to the service user's home. Service user(1)'s needs are classed as 'social care', as she does not require regular medical input.

Service user(1) prefers holistic assessment to the previous system, in which various practitioners assessed needs related only to their own area of work. Service user(1) spoke about it being 'intrusive', as it entailed so many people visiting her home. She felt 'not threatened, that's too strong a word; but it's your own territory'. The number of people coming in and out was very 'disruptive'.

Before her husband died, they were receiving visits from home care assistants, and district nurses came three times a week, as her husband required regular medical input. Service user(1) described the district nurses as 'for want of a better word, very nosy – they can rule your life'.

Service user(1) is happier now, where it is mutually agreed between her and the social worker whether any particular practitioner needs to visit. 'She wouldn't dare send someone in without asking permission; they'd get very short shrift.'

The direct payment system allows service users a great deal of leeway to organize their own services. Under this system, the service user becomes the employer and so has to assume the accompanying obligations. So this is 'not all plain sailing. You have to take responsibility, you've got to hire and fire.' Service user(1) attends to the training needs of her personal assistants (PAs), and will send them on courses should they require particular skills, for example manual handling.

The direct payments system is brokered through a Centre for Inclusive Living (CIL), which was started in 1994 by six people with disabilities. Service user(1) was involved with its early development and she is also involved with other organizations to develop services. She started receiving direct payments in 2000; before that she was in receipt of home care, which she found too structured for her needs. The team leader told the home care workers what they could do and Service user(1) had very little say in the care they provided. For example she couldn't even have a bath every day. She is much happier employing PAs herself: 'They do what I tell them.' She advertises on employment websites when she needs a new PA.

To illustrate the lack of flexibility in the home care system, Service user(1) related what had happened when she recently lost one of her PAs. The ACC service helped her with emergency cover, arranging for an agency worker to visit her for two nights. Service user(1) said the agency worker was a 'very nice young lady', but she arrived at 7.30 p.m., and only had half an hour with her. During this time, the worker needed to cook a meal, help Service user(1) to eat it, and then help her get to bed. Service user(1) almost choked in bed, as the whole process had been so rushed. She chose to sit up in her wheelchair for the whole of the second night, rather than be rushed in this way.

Discussion with a carer

'People have left my mother with a sense of a lack of dignity; she felt quite violated . . . sometimes they used to talk over her, she was deaf and partially sighted and they wouldn't give her time to speak in her own language. They spoke for her: "Oh, I see, what you are saying is . . . " and I would say "No! She's not saying that at all! Listen to her." It's all tied up with dignity and respect, listening to people and not being prescriptive.

People have come into my home at different times . . . as a carer I've had a lack of respect, lack of consideration, prescriptive behaviour . . . I had applied for a lift . . . and the person said, "Well that will have to go and . . . can you take that out to so and so." I was standing there and I said, "Hey, what about me? You know, I live here too."

The single assessment process as I understood it was designed to enable the first person in to garner as much information as possible so that the second person didn't come in after and ask the same questions, because that was something that was so infuriating having to answer the same questions over and over.'

Workers in the voluntary sector

Community development worker

'I'll give the proper definition of what the voluntary sector is, because most people, almost everybody, including in the voluntary sector, they don't understand it, they think it's made up of volunteers, or whatever. What it means is that the statutory sector is legislated, so that it *has* to provide some services by law; the voluntary sector is those bodies who pick up areas which don't, by law, have to be covered, but which they can see are absolutely essential and vital to the wellbeing of people; that's the voluntary bit, so that's at the heart of what we do. And I think it behoves people to understand that, because we're not a bunch of volunteers – although there are lots of volunteers involved, and of course management committees, trustees of organizations, are all volunteers, and we're not for profit; but it doesn't make us third-rate or amateurish. Our voluntary bit is that we've decided that something is absolutely vital, and therefore we will raise the money and get the workforce to do something about it.
. . .
We started off with a survey of what did people think that *town* needed and wanted, that broke down to the needs of older people, children, young people and families, traffic and transport issues, environmental issues . . . year by year, we've concentrated on one area and then another . . . We try and improve services and facilities within those different areas . . . we're often working in big partnership groups often across the whole of *county*. With older people, we were one of the people involved in getting a permanent care and repair organization that covers *county*, where people can get practical help, and get

their houses repaired if they're on low incomes . . . Loneliness, that's why we started our Contact the Elderly group, which is a monthly outing to tea for elderly people who live alone and are housebound . . .

I, over the last twelve years, have sat on a whole series of review boards, which have looked at local authority strategies and policies on various aspects of community care that affect older people, including things like day care and home care and where you set the threshold to receive services . . . currently I'm sitting on this Older People's Programme group which is meant to oversee every single programme and strategy . . . I'm representing the voluntary sector across the whole of *county*, not just my group.'

'What's your experience been like working with different professionals and statutory bodies?'

'I think I'm in a very advantageous position, because my background is in architecture; and architecture is, in a way, the essence of partnership working . . . everyone is equal at the table and treated as a professional; but also you get used to dealing with fairly high-powered partnership situations . . . that's quite a good background in a lot of ways for doing what I'm doing now, I'm not easily intimidated, I make a point of not minding to ask stupid questions; because also I know very well that most people . . . who think they're very high-powered have got very limited and narrow knowledge, if they step outside that they actually don't know very much at all . . . People from the different professions have been told so often that they're supposed to be working with the community, or working with the voluntary sector, so they do try their best; and if they fail and you pick them up on it, they tend to try and improve things; but there is often, especially with health, the NHS . . . they try and smooth things over and carry on regardless.

. . . there's been an awful lot of consultation for the sake of it . . . in directives from the government down, it does say that consultation has to be meaningful, and you don't just get people to state an opinion and then ignore it entirely, what people say is meant to change policy . . . it's generally moving in the right direction; . . . it's so built-in to policy directives now, people have had to learn more and more how to deal constructively with the voluntary sector.

The . . . Older People's Programme group...there's twenty people round a room, there may be three or four of us from the voluntary sector . . . local authority and health . . . a representative from care homes. . . . I find myself piping up a lot and saying, "What does that mean?", and it'll turn out that quite a lot of other people in the room won't know what it means either; because they're coming from different disciplines, so they will sneak up to you afterwards and say, "I'm glad you asked that question." But I think it's maybe surprising how many of them wouldn't have . . .

. . . what I've found myself doing is always trying to couch things in terms of constructive suggestions, not saying, "Oh, it's so awful" and "Why don't you do this?" and "Why have you done that?", but saying, "From now on, would it be possible to do this?", just to keep any ruffled feathers smoothed over. I was at one meeting where, after every single item, I had a big point to make, and I said, "Oh God, you must be sick of the sound of my voice now" – and they all went, "No, no, no, no, it's fine, it's jolly interesting, glad to hear from you" . . . I do have quite a broad perspective, and they do seem to miss off whole views of how the ordinary person on the ground takes these things . . . '

'What are the mechanics of actually working with different bodies and organizations?'

'I don't know that it's anything more than meetings and paper. The usual thing, you get reports, you read reports, you underline things in red, you go to meetings, raise questions, and those get minuted, in however legible or illegible a form, and then on to the next thing. Those meetings and those reports are the means of communication . . . '

'What do you think the key issues are for the voluntary sector in relation to the statutory sector?'

'They are treated unfairly . . . an awful lot of the work that gets done doesn't raise any revenue, and therefore to do it, you're dependent on grants; and an awful lot of the most important grants come from local authorities . . . they think they're marvellous now to have got up to three-year funding. It's surprising how quick three years will go whizzing by . . . there is still one-year funding that goes on... to do any core or ongoing work, is an absolute battle; it shouldn't be like that . . . to get the money for it is often so difficult . . . often the basis on which, for instance, social services commission stuff from a voluntary organization is not on a level playing field, a commercial organization will get away with masses more than a voluntary organization, which may be tied down with all sorts of really unfair conditions . . . and the local authority seems to think it's OK for it to suddenly change the complete brief on which someone's tendered . . .

There's these things called compacts . . . something that the government has really enforced on all local authorities to produce. It's a voluntary agreement between statutory organizations and the voluntary sector, including social economy organizations, that is, ones that earn money but are still not for profit; and they take forever to develop, and there's big partnerships involved . . . the idea is that both sides have rights and responsibilities . . . it covers a whole spectrum . . . not just to do with where you're receiving money or grants from them. A lot of it's about how you [local authorities] consult with the community and voluntary organizations, how you don't abuse them in consultations, one of the main things being you just use them as tick-boxes but ignore what they say, so you simply abuse all their time and energy as although it didn't count for anything . . .

What makes [the voluntary sector] such a great place to work in . . . is that it's got this terrific can-do attitude . . . you get a bunch of people together, and you raise some money, and you campaign and you get policies changed, laws changed and attitudes changed from the bottom right up to government level; and you get something in place that didn't exist before, that no one else was going to pay for, but everybody was crying out for the need of it . . . whereas often, in local authorities for instance . . . you are enmeshed in such a net of restrictive codes and protocols. We can do things with money . . . with so much greater freedom than someone in a parish council, or a local authority, or a PCT . . . no matter how much they try and free up budgets, it's amazing how restrictive budgetary rules are, and how much it can stop people doing. So there's that sort of freshness, that freedom, that vitality there, that response to what's actually needed, rather than the theory, or something from ten years ago. Even if you don't succeed entirely, the failure's probably got a lot of good things about it.

The worst thing about it is probably this short-termism, where you see wonderful things started, and then have the plug pulled on them; and you know that they've done so much good, so many people wanted them, and now they've just disappeared again; it took so much effort to set it up, and now you may never see anything like it again . . . a statutory organization is budgeted, it can always only do so much, then you see these painful gaps it leaves, and you do your best for those, but often you can't do enough, long enough.'

Manager in a large voluntary agency

'What involvement did you have with strategic developments?'

'As an Assistant Director I was on a couple of Children's Trusts connected with developing a strategic Children's Plan, doing analysis of local provision and preparing for inspections...The other people involved were mainly statutory sector people and there tended to only be one representative of the big and one representative of the small vollies [voluntary agencies]... There were different levels of buy-in, some people had to be involved as part of their jobs, for others even if they wanted to be involved there were questions about how much time they had and how it could be resourced, since, unlike the statutory sector, the voluntary sector is not automatically resourced to be involved in local strategic developments. I tried to support people from the smaller voluntaries that were often close to users and had user representation, to help them get funding from the Trust to participate and be involved . . . Another factor was that some Trust members had quite boundaried roles, others had more autonomy, others were not able to make any decisions and had to take things back for further consultation. This could make things quite cumbersome.

In one Children's Trust I had lead responsibility . . . for developing its participation strategy for children and their families and carers. There are challenges around the area of children's involvement. Different professional groups have very different understanding, experiences and attitudes around participation and there can be tensions around this. There are some people who have probably done a lot around participation, for example youth workers and the development of youth parliaments, but they are dealing with the older end and they are also not necessarily stitched in to what is happening to children and young people in education. There, the emphasis is on school councils . . . these can end up as representing the best-behaved pupils and there is lots of research around pupil voice that indicates that this is an area that needs much more development . . . Then there are groups who want to engage younger children, and sometimes it is quite hard for professionals who work with older age groups to acknowledge the competence that younger children have and not to think that older children should always be the representatives. The interprofessional debates can also have a gender element as there are more men in youth work and more women working with younger children. With disabled children there is a tradition of quite a lot of parent involvement as well as child involvement, and then you have issues about how to manage that and how to effectively engage children and young people with complex needs.

Parents made up half of the management board of the Sure Start local programme; I think this was an easier strategy to effect because a voluntary agency was the accountable body. We also tried to develop as many opportunities as possible to get parents involved in training and to employ local people. For example, we created posts like family support workers, midwife assistants and speech and language assistants, as well as volunteer posts such as Breastfeeding Babes supporters. Family support workers were established from the outset; the others were negotiated . . . once the programme was up and running, inter-agency trust had been established . . . '

'*What about collaboration at Sure Start project level?*'

'This varied quite a lot. Relationships could be quite fragile so they needed a lot of nurturing, if you get reluctant professionals this can be very difficult to turn round. Sometimes it's difficult to pinpoint what the issues are. For example, we worked with two health centres, both had been involved in developing the Sure Start proposal, yet there was quite a difference in their approach and level of engagement although they were working for the same health trust with the same managers. Some things are about individuals, some things about informal leadership and the way people were supervised and their accountability structures, these vary a lot between different professionals.

There were issues for speech and language therapists, as sometimes they were asked to approach things in a way that they had not been trained for. In one project it was important for them to train and support all staff to have a basic level of skills in recognizing speech and language problems and to know how to refer for more specialist help, but also able to encourage all children's speech and language development to as high a level as possible . . . initially they found it challenging to work out what was good enough for an early-years worker . . . Another thing they were asked to do was to be available to provide advice on a regular drop-in basis to any parent who wanted it . . . here they were asked just to respond to unexpected situations . . . This could be challenging, I don't think they were being defensive, but this was out of their territory. On the one hand, they were used to more longer-term clinical interventions with people with more complex problems . . . What Sure Start was asking of them was much lower down the system, just trying to raise the level of speech and language skills in the whole community. They would like to have been able to offer more intensive support in some situations but that was not what parents were asking for at that time. These were some of the issues about self-referral and user participation that were challenging . . . '

'What about social workers; did they feel that other disciplines were potentially stepping on their toes or issues about their role that they found challenging?'

'There was considerable 'in principle' support from the local social services managers but this was not necessarily seen as a priority at more senior levels, so social services' strategic participation [for example, on the management board] was quite limited. At an operational level there were issues to be resolved around child protection . . . when referrals should be made, how you get a response . . . confidentiality, service user involvement . . . what sort of services people are offered – by and large local authority social workers are not that well stitched in to what is going on in communities, and I think they probably under-use the resources that are there mainly because they don't know enough about them or enough to trust them.'

'How did confidentially issues get resolved?'

'Different tactics really, clear guidelines on how to make referrals . . . we identified link people like duty team managers who would understand where the agency was coming from. Also training, going to social work team meetings, mutual information-sharing . . . we had a system where at inter-agency team meetings people took it in turns to talk about their roles and it was open to anyone working or funded by Sure Start to participate. Different professions would take the agenda for half an hour and share what they thought others needed to know about their service and interprofessional or inter-agency dilemmas and issues. As a lot of the para-professionals were local parents, this was a really good opportunity for capacity building.'

'What about user involvement, I know this was really important – did anyone take the lead on establishing that, or was it accepted in the philosophy of the projects?'

'Yes, in the philosophy, so it made it much easier for us to do and we took it very seriously. The management board had equal numbers of 'parent manager' and agency representatives, and we developed a parent-led forum at each 'site', so there was a considerable degree of user control rather than just user involvement. We worked very hard at capacity building, which raised lots of fascinating issues . . . what people in a local area should know about other people in the local area . . . There are also issues about skills sets and skills development . . . we felt that whatever energy we put into local capacity building and training, the benefits should go back into the local community rather than leaving it each evening as non-local staff drive home. We had very good success with that. This type of involvement may take longer to reap benefits and some other types of involvement may look better on the surface, and give quicker immediate returns. I think the national Sure Start research shows that you need both good, professionally skilled leadership, properly trained, keeping an eye on standards and supporting quality along with local staff to

achieve the best from capacity building, because then what you get in is a real buy-in and a real appreciation from the community that it is for them.'
. . .

'What about issues in terms of tensions between medical and social models around projects in relation to disabled children?'

'One area of potential tension was around inclusive structures and inclusive groups. We dealt with this by having some early-years workers looking at what the problems were and then trying to deal with it. So the early years staff had special training with educational psychologists and specialist social workers for disabled children. We also trained up some staff to create peripatetic posts, not just to accompany a disabled child into an inclusive early-years setting but to make that setting and everything about it, including staff, suitable, so that the child was really included and the parents happy. This was very important for parents . . . '

'Where you were able to be creative, did you feel that the interprofessional context made a difference?'

'Yes, for sure. When people felt valued for their knowledge that was important. Also for many people in specialist roles there are not many colleagues about in a local area and it can be quite lonely. If people didn't work well together they would always be arriving into settings where they didn't know anyone, rather than arriving in places where people knew them and made them feel welcome . . . Also, when staff from one setting had an idea that they wanted to see implemented, it was often very helpful to have interprofessional back-up in arguing for that within their agency, and of course we were also able to access parents and children's views to add to the evidence.'

'It sounds like a lot of the relationships evolved and were worked through . . . '

'Relationships with the midwives were very positive; I think that was partly about the personalities and skills of those involved but also it helped to have a midwife funded directly by Sure Start and seconded to the programme . . .

Health visitors were key to a successful Sure Start programme, since they are the people who best know families with young children in the area and, after word of mouth, the people most likely to introduce families . . . therefore their individual commitment was very important and most were supportive and engaged. However, health visitors were in a very difficult position, they had been told their role was changing. They had huge caseloads . . . the number of universal visits have been cut, they are supposed to concentrate on children in need and have an increased role around parenting skills *but* the way the medical model works is that they have a huge amount of autonomy in the sort of training they take on, how they plan their work and what they take on . . . This meant that they carried a lot of anxiety around child-protection issues . . . Many of them were very unhappy with these developments and felt very angry that their families were not being looked after. They wanted to do universal visits and spend more time with families in need and felt that the service was not funded sufficiently to use their skills to best advantage . . . they seemed to have much less case and workload supervision than social workers commonly have. They were the most disaffected group in my experience and the group that found it most difficult to come to a common view about their role, which led to internal and inter-agency difficulties.

They also seemed to have very different polices and expectations in relation to inter-agency collaboration...looking at some health-visitor training guidelines from the Department of Health, I was really surprised that it said the HV [health visitor] role is to be *the* lead professional around early years and to make things happen in their locality, to instruct other people . . . there was no mention of partnership or collaboration . . . It gave the strong view that they were the only leaders, the people who ran the show for early years. Regardless of Sure Start, that approach did not take enough account of other early-years services, or of service users, and was impossible due to their caseload, but at one level they were being given that message . . . Most were involved in some sort of group work, even although there were lots of demands on their time. But it was challenging for many programmes because they were more used to the autonomy of deciding amongst themselves, or on an individual basis, what type of initiative they would pursue.'

Other professionals

Health visitor

'I worked very closely with the NCH [National Children's Home], because they had a building adjacent to the clinic . . . we set up various groups together, which worked very well. Home-Start is another one that I've worked with quite closely, Barnardo's . . . Some individual charities, like for a particular condition, like MS [multiple sclerosis] or cancer, or whatever, referring and linking in with those, if I've got a client or a family with a particular problem or disease . . . I find information from there, or get links in to them.

They're normally very good at giving information, giving advice, welcoming contact from the family, but it just takes time. That's the only negative thing. I've found libraries have been superb . . . they're very good at giving advice about where to go for what, and it's also a way of getting people into a library.

The Sure Start areas were set up with user involvement right in the beginning as what they were going to do with the money, how it was going to be set up, etcetera. So the idea for Sure Start is that it's, not come from the community necessarily, but there's been heavy involvement . . . With the children's centres now, I would be quite surprised if there's been any user involvement, what I call true user involvement, because they've really been imposed on particular areas, rather than areas saying, "Oh, we really want a children's centre" [a community centre where all the relevant services are under one roof, along with other spaces such as a café].

It's quite difficult for health visitors to know what their actual role is, because there're people coming in saying, "Well, I can do this bit." Then you've got the voluntary sector doing, well, they're doing parenting courses.

Health visitors thought that parenting was part of their remit, and it is . . . but now there are a lot of voluntary organizations doing some sort of parenting, emotional, relationship, whatever it might be, and health visitors have generally felt really quite insecure about where they're meant to be going.'

GP

'We are much more aware of who is caring for whom; and patient confidentiality is important here. There is a great temptation at times to talk to the carer rather than patient. So you always have to remember who is the patient. Carers are marked up on the database, we are aware of their needs, and that they are not taking other jobs and get carers' allowances, so you have to make sure you support them.'

Senior registrar, paediatrics

'I always treat children as I would treat an adult, although the words you use sometimes are different. The longer that a child has been in the system, the more generally they understand. So someone with cancer who's been diagnosed at two will know an awful lot about their disease by the time they get to four or five, and they'll be probably be Gillick-competent[1] by the time they get to six or seven, maybe. So they've had four years of treatment and they're on their second bone-marrow transplant; you should listen to them, if they say, "Listen, I'm not sure I want to do this again" . . . they would have a very good understanding . . . and the parents equally would have a very good understanding, and you could have a much more educated discussion with them.

I think doctors give a lot of information. I was just talking to a consultant this morning, and she was talking, when I said, "How do you interact with the service users?" She kept describing information she was giving, she wants the patient apparently to fit in with our agenda, on the basis that if you do as we tell you, you'll get better, so if you take your treatments properly, if you have this kind of diet, if you do these things. I didn't hear a lot about, "What are you looking for from the service, and how can we make it better?" I think the emerging thinking is all about changing to fit in with the desires and needs of families and users, rather than us telling them what they should be doing . . . '

Summary

The voices of service users, carers and voluntary (third-sector) workers remind us why effective working together is important. The increasing use of direct payments and services provided by non-statutory services reflects the difficulties the statutory services can experience when trying to provide personalized care that meets the needs of individuals.

REFLECTIVE ACTIVITY

After reading the diverse views in this chapter, reflect on what you have learned about how undertaking professional education can limit as well as deepen understanding of public, community and individual health.

Alternative services, however, have their own problems with providing care and support.

Make a list of the difficulties identified by contributors to this chapter. Take time to reflect on what you have learned about the importance of user involvement in planning and providing services. Review your observations after you have read each chapter in Part II.

Note

1 If a child (16 years or younger) has Gillick competence, it means that he/she is considered to possess enough understanding to be able to consent to his/her own medical treatment, without the need for parental permission or knowledge.

Maternity and Infant Care

Material collated by
Katherine C Pollard

In this chapter, we present excerpts from staff working in an NHS maternity unit, as well as from three women who received care from the unit staff. All these individuals were interviewed for a research study exploring midwives' interprofessional relationships (Pollard 2007). The researcher also spent time observing interprofessional interaction in the unit.

The unit comprised a delivery suite, a ward and an antenatal clinic. Women were admitted to the delivery suite in labour, and were transferred to the ward after they had given birth. Women would also be admitted to the ward if experiencing medical problems during pregnancy. Staff generally considered interprofessional working to be good, with some caveats concerning specific staff–group interactions. There were question marks about the degree to which women using the service were included in processes of care co-ordination and decision-making.

Service scenario 1

Clinical practice in NHS maternity units is governed by locally determined policies and protocols. In the first two excerpts, midwives are asked their opinion of two unit policies, one concerning labour, the other the administration of Vitamin K, a substance involved in blood-clotting. There can be differences between midwifery and medical perspectives when assessing labour progress. This arises from the different stances which the professions take:

generally speaking, obstetricians rely on precise measurement of specific physiological processes in relation to strict time points; midwives, however, usually rely on an overview of these same processes, within a more flexible time-frame (Silverton 1993). Newborn babies have comparatively low levels of Vitamin K, and the Department of Health recommends that all babies be given Vitamin K shortly after birth (DH 1998). It is commonly midwives who tell parents about this, and who give babies Vitamin K, usually by injection.

Senior midwife: delivery suite

' . . . we've got a good relationship with the obstetric physios [physiotherapists], we've got a good relationship with the obstetric staff [medical house officers, registrars and consultants]; theatre, pretty good . . . and with NICU [neonatal intensive care unit] as well . . . everybody has their differences of opinions, and certainly you'll meet personalities that don't like personalities, but as groups of professionals, I think it's probably about as good as it's been anywhere I've ever worked . . .

. . . there's good communication between everybody. I think that the obstetric staff have a certain amount of respect for the midwives and vice versa . . . most midwives enjoy working as midwives here because it's a pretty laid-back set-up, and midwives certainly are given their full autonomy . . . we don't have a situation which other units have, where the registrars try to do ward rounds three times a day . . . actually going into labour rooms . . . The senior midwife will co-ordinate with the reg [registrar] and they'll go into rooms if they're invited . . . I think that engenders a lot of respect by the midwives, because they don't feel that someone's coming in and chasing them; but they also know because no one's coming in, they have to think for themselves. I think the midwives work well together, and there's good liaison between senior midwives and the registrars . . . because people are allowed to work within their full scope it makes them happier in what they're doing professionally, and I think that helps. It just seems to be very friendly, and I think we're very lucky like that . . . we're in the middle of NICU and theatres, and the obstetric physios work over here, so I think from that point of view we're quite central; and I think people work hard to keep those relationships going as well, I think there is a lot of input from a lot of people in order to make sure that those relationships don't break down too often; and if there are problems with relationships between various professional groups that they're addressed rather than being allowed to ferment into a bigger problem . . . '

' . . . *occasionally there's obviously a slight difference of clinical opinion between the midwifery staff and the obstetric staff . . . ?*'

' . . . I think it does happen, and I think that's a good thing, anyway, because as a rule it keeps everybody thinking . . . a large majority of our registrars, if you say to them . . . "I'm not totally convinced about this, what do you think?", they're very happy to discuss it; and certainly the consultants, you can say to them, "Well, this is what I think, what do you think?" There have been a couple of occasions where I've had to call a consultant over the head of a registrar and say, "I'm not happy with your decision, if you're not prepared to discuss it with me I'm going to call the consultant", and on those two occasions I've had excellent response from the consultant, who's been prepared to come in and talk to us both and sort it out . . . as a midwife your responsibility is to go to the highest authority to deal with it, if you don't feel comfortable; but generally we've managed to resolve most things without having to get anybody else involved, but if you have to call a consultant, you have to call a consultant.'

. . .

'. . . *in one of the [unit] labour policies, a labour that's progressing at less than a centimetre an hour is defined as being primarily dysfunctional . . . ?*'

'I don't think it's a totally reasonable definition . . . I think we all know as midwives that sometimes people just aren't progressing to that full amount but you know that they're progressing . . . but you've got to have a guide, and I think it's reasonable to have a guide for what functional labour and dysfunctional labour is, because otherwise you will end up with those situations where suddenly, someone's been very slow in labour for a very long time . . . I think there's always room for negotiation. It's very unusual, and I've certainly never been in the situation myself where a registrar has bombastically said, "No, you must do this"; if you say, "Look, just give me two hours, I'm really sure things are changing here" . . . the definition is harsh, but I think there has to be something in this litigious age, I think it's very reasonable in an obstetric unit to have a definition like that, because I think that otherwise there's too much room for people not taking action.'

'*The NVQ [National Vocational Qualification] training for the HCAs [health care assistants/nursing auxiliaries], doing blood pressures and things like that . . . ?*'

'. . . anything that can be done to relieve the clinical burden, or the burden of midwives, so they can be allowed to do their clinical midwifery can only be a good thing. I think doing it in a structured way, like NVQ with midwives teaching and assessing the NAs [nursing auxiliaries], has got to be a good thing . . . I really believe that we need to be looking at resources like NAs with NVQ training to do stuff that you don't need a trained midwife to do, because otherwise this profession's going to collapse within the NHS . . .

. . . I'm not trying to say this is a perfect environment, because it isn't, but . . . I think this is a very friendly place . . . the support of the obstetricians, the support of the consultants . . . I think that's why the structure does work well, because [the senior midwives] feel supported and they can therefore support the junior midwives . . . I think that we're doing the best that we can, I think we're doing a good job . . . '

Community midwife(1)

'*I notice the very last thing on the Vitamin K policy says that if a woman refuses Vitamin K she should be referred to a paediatrician; and I just wondered what you felt about that?*'

'I agree with that. We have to try and give information in a very unbiased way, and with as much medical knowledge, I suppose, behind what information we're giving as possible; and, you know, things are moving on all the time in terms of research, and although we try and keep up to date, I do feel sometimes the paediatricians could be more up to date than we are; and I also know [a paediatric consultant] in particular is very happy to speak to parents if they've decided they don't want to give Vitamin K, for whatever reasons; and I feel the parents don't always have the full information and knowledge at their fingertips to make a decision, and so I do feel somebody even more in the know than me can still give them unbiased information, if you like . . . to help them make a decision, help them make a choice.'

Service scenario 2

In the next two excerpts, among other issues, consultant obstetricians speak about midwives in the unit being ventouse practitioners. It is unusual to find midwives, rather than obstetricians, conducting ventouse deliveries, which entail the extraction of the baby from the mother's vagina by means of a mechanized vacuum device (Silverton 1993).

Obstetric consultant(1) (male)

'We've got a very good team of midwives here, a very professional group, and we link in with them on a regular basis on labour ward with the management of patients. We have occasionally had situations where junior staff [obstetricians] have perhaps been inexperienced and haven't always come up with the right kind of decision on a situation, and the midwives always know they can phone the consultant on call and explain the issue, and we need to assess the situation ourselves, so there's that sort of thing. Occasionally there are social events, you know, and that always I think helps with team building . . .

. . . because of 'Changing Childbirth',[1] doctors not being part of the primary care-givers in labour, and with it being more midwifery-led, the GPs by and large have become less and less interested in intrapartum [labour] care, and the newer recruits to general practice . . . have tended not to want to maintain an intrapartum management presence so it's [the ventouse] been very much devolved to the midwives; the midwives have therefore been skilled up to provide a level of care that previously wasn't available . . . '

Obstetric consultant(2) (female)

'I think it's really good, actually . . . I've worked here off and on for almost fifteen years now. So I started at a sort of middle-grade level and came back as a registrar, then a senior registrar, and now at consultant level . . . there is a good atmosphere by and large, everybody's friendly, most people are on first-name terms . . . we occasionally get the odd problem with a newish junior doctor, often male, [laughs] who insists on treating the midwives as nurses to do exactly as he tells them, as the doctor; but it's never the kind of permanent staff that are here, you know, we do not tolerate that, and we say to our juniors, the midwives know far more than you guys know, and you must respect them and defer to them, they're professionals in their own right . . .

. . . traditionally this [geographical] area has allowed women perhaps more choice than other areas and therefore midwives more autonomy, so there's never in this region been a concept that the midwives are only there to help the obstetricians, I think it's always been felt that midwives are there to be the professional looking after normal pregnancy, normal labour . . . there is definitely a feeling that they're not just adjuncts to obstetricians . . . and that pregnancy isn't necessarily an obstetrician's remit all the time . . . I think we do manage to work quite well in parallel . . . midwives have their area of expertise, hopefully we've got our area of expertise and we can work together and not actually feel threatened by either side . . . '

'The fact that midwives do ventouse deliveries, what effect do you think that's had on the relationships between the obstetricians and the midwives?'

'I think it's probably helped even more to make the doctors appreciate that . . . they are highly skilled professionals . . . there is always, of course, the slight worry that our most junior middle grades lose out a little bit of experience . . . but I don't think that's been a major problem, 'cos the criteria for when a midwife can do it are really quite strict . . . I think there's enough here for everybody, and I think people are just really pleased if they've got a midwife ventouse practitioner on with them, because they actually see that person as being much more their kind of key helper than, for example, the junior doctor who runs around, but can't actually get the women delivered, so I don't think it's been a problem, I think it's helped our perception of midwives, if anything.'

'You've got this system where midwives are assisting in theatre . . . ?'

'That came about because we don't have enough junior doctors to provide adequate cover in the middle of the night . . . or to provide it within the confines of the European Working Time Directive,[2] we actually were doing fine until we had to reduce the length of hours that our juniors could be in hospital . . . '

'I've noticed that most [interaction] seems to occur between obstetricians and the senior midwives?'

'That's probably true. I guess we know them better because they've been around longer . . . when you go to do your ward round, when you take on your on-call shift . . . it's the senior midwife who will . . . take you through what's going on on the entire labour ward . . . I usually ask to speak to . . . .the G grade [senior midwife] who's in charge of the shift because I expect them to know about all the rooms as opposed to just the ladies that have been allocated to them . . . some of the people who aren't G grades because they're only part-time, but have nevertheless been around for a long time, I think we probably think of them in the same breath as we would the G grades. . . . if you've got a student midwife, or a newly qualified midwife, particularly if she starts off working on one of the wards where I don't normally have patients, then I wouldn't get to know her name quite so quickly . . . it probably goes both ways . . . when they just start they may be shyer of coming up to us directly, until they get to know us better so they may actually go through the G grades as well . . .

. . . it obviously makes sense for the senior midwife to know where the registrar is . . . it's better if she knows, "OK, this is the priority, this is where I want him to go first and when he's finished that, I'll send him into the other room to do whatever's there"; so I think it's to make it . . . the whole system work better . . . the registrar can't co-ordinate it because they're not physically present on the labour ward all the time, so it's got to be co-ordinated by the . . . midwife in charge of the shift . . .

. . . [the midwives] work very well with the anaesthetists . . . I think there's a lot of respect on both sides . . . I'm horrified to hear how it doesn't work so well in other units. And occasionally they [the midwives] say, "It's extraordinary, you let us do this or let us do that", and I just think, "Of course." . . . [midwife] in the antenatal clinic . . . knows so much about foetal medicine its kind of crazy not to use that expertise . . . anybody who can contribute anything, it's all gratefully received and that's fine, 'cos we all . . . want as many healthy women and healthy babies as possible, so it's a good, fun unit to work in.'

Service scenario 3

In the next excerpt, an obstetric registrar mentions her expertise in interpreting foetal heart monitor recordings. During pregnancy and labour, babies' well-being is assessed by means of a foetal heart monitor (Silverton 1993).

Obstetric registrar (female)

'It's quite easy to be intimidated by one or two of those senior midwives because obviously they've been there, done that, for the last thirty years; but their appreciation has to be that at the end of the day they're not the doctor, so the buck doesn't stop with them, it stops with us . . . it's us who's done the delivery. So there's give and take on both sides, there is respect for both, I think. . . . there can be some intimidation between some of their senior staff and some questioning from that point of view . . . it depends on how you work on one particular shift. I think the power generally is evenly shared . . . everyone interacts well with each other and asks opinions . . . it's not "doctor knows best", it is about opinions . . . the midwife may have seen it a hundred times, I may never have come across it before. It's about asking and sharing information; but there are also situations where because the midwife has seen a situation similar to that in how many years that the potential is for a junior registrar to feel intimidated by that, and possibly go with the midwife's decision rather than the decision you feel that you should be taking.

. . . most of the senior midwives are going to be a lot more experienced in their career than I ever will be at normal midwifery . . . but I will always be more experienced than them in instrumental deliveries and caesarean sections and bad traces [foetal heart monitor readings] and those sorts of things that the doctor's called for . . . I think as long as people realize that that's where their role is invaluable . . . within the realm of normal, and our role is invaluable within the realm of abnormal labour, and as long as we work together and both recognize that we're both there for the patients, it shouldn't be a jealousy thing . . . There has to be some appreciation that we're both needed, midwives are needed, doctors are needed.'

Service scenario 4

The next excerpt concerns a woman with Rhesus-negative blood. To prevent possible problems in future pregnancies, women whose blood type is Rhesus negative are offered a substance called anti-D during pregnancy. Should the baby's blood type be Rhesus-positive, women are also offered anti-D after they have given birth (Silverton 1993).

Service user(2)

'They said, "Well, what we do under the NICE [National Institute of Clinical Excellence] guidelines . . . you will get three doses of anti-D . . . the first time I went to have it done, I turned up at the doctor's surgery as normal for my antenatal appointment, I said, "Oh, I've come for my anti-D today", she looked at me, "We don't do it here" . . . they had forgotten to book me in, I had to go to a hospital, so I rushed to the hospital next morning . . . waited over half an hour, and nobody brought it over, they were arguing amongst themselves over who should have brought it from the different department . . . it went to the pharmacy and nobody brought it back over . . . The second time . . . absolutely brilliant, turned up to my appointment, midwife was there, gave me my injection, absolutely fab, brilliant, no problem at all . . .

. . . I kept saying to the midwife, while I was giving birth, "Don't forget my anti-D" and . . . once again when I got upstairs [to the ward] I mentioned anti-D, and the grumpy midwife looked at me and said, "Oh I don't think that's necessary" . . . and of course it turned out the second day she gave it to me . . .

. . . it's just [sighs], the community midwives are saying, "Oh yes, this is a standard procedure" . . . as soon as you go upstairs, "Well, it might not be necessary, we don't know" and in the end they gave it to me anyway . . . '

Service scenario 5

Under English law, women have the right to choose where they give birth. Maternity professionals can recommend a particular place of birth, but normally have no power to enforce that recommendation. Midwives are not allowed to withdraw care, even if they disagree with a woman's decision regarding the place of birth (NMC 2004). Women also have the right to decide whether or not to accept care for themselves and their babies.

Service user(3): had her baby at home

'The community midwife measured my bump and it seemed smaller so she said, "I can't just let it go" . . . I had the [hospital] appointment in the morning, we ended up being there for about seven hours . . . I had this appointment with the consultant but he was too busy to see me at the right time so I had to see the midwife first . . . she took my blood pressure and saw it was through the roof and went off and got him and he did, we were supposed to be checking the size of my bump, he essentially actually said, "Well it quite often happens around this stage because the baby engages, the bump gets smaller" . . . but then obviously waiting on the blood-test results and he'd gone and we had another midwife . . . and then I got strapped on to the foetal heart monitor . . . and then somebody else came along and midwife [number] four came along and took us off to the lounge where we proceeded to sit for five hours or something, waiting for blood-test results . . . '

'*Then the SHO [Senior House Officer] came . . . ?*'

'Yes, with another midwife, number five . . . they then explained to me why it would be a great thing, in fact they weren't really explaining to me why it would be a great thing if I got induced, they were explaining to me why they were going to induce me essentially . . . '

'*Did you get that sense coming from both of them?*'

'Yes, oh absolutely, they were stood very close, stood up as well, I was sitting down . . . my partner, at first he'd been like sort of, "I don't really like this whole home birth idea, I'd much rather you were somewhere safe" – he was utterly swayed towards home birth just by that experience in the hospital . . . I think it was the way they didn't say, "Can we induce you please?", "Would you consent to being induced?", "We want to induce you tomorrow, so . . . " – it was very brusque and businesslike and, "Let's get on with the arrangements" [clicks fingers] rather than taking me through benefits, risks, alternatives, maybe, a bit more explanation as to why it would be necessary, do I have any questions . . . it was almost like, "You're ours now, we can do what we like and that's it, you're here", almost, rather than working with, you know, somebody who's clearly heavily pregnant, clearly quite upset . . . '

Service user(4): labour induced owing to medical problems

'We went into the hospital that evening and they monitored us and tried to convince me to stay in and I also have two small children at home I wasn't keen on that . . . [the obstetric registrar] just wasn't communicative and wasn't able to understand that we might not be keen on having a scan or doing a test or doing this and that, staying in hospital, he just seemed to think that whatever he suggested ought to be exactly what we did . . . the midwife was useful when she came back after he'd gone . . . she was quite good at sitting down and explaining what she thought was going on, so it was good and bad . . . she was very supportive, she said it was fine [to go home] . . . '

'*What was your overall impression of the quality of the communication between the community midwives and the hospital team?*'

' . . . the midwife-to-midwife communication seemed good, the [community] team midwives communicating with the [obstetric and paediatric] registrars seemed sometimes to be difficult . . . my impression was that the team midwives, because they're much more intimately involved in the patients . . . know what our preferences are; and when they deal with the registrars who simply say, "Look, this is how we do it, you just need to do this this way, whether there's a good reason for it or not" . . . she found that frustrating because I know she had tried to lobby to allow us to go home straight after the baby was born . . . but they [the paediatricians] were just adamant that they weren't going to let him go . . .

. . . [the midwife] was quite keen for us to go home if that was what we wanted, to the point of going and speaking to them [the paediatricians] even although she suspected that it would be difficult to get that arranged . . . but I don't think that she ever was able to sort of sway them, if her opinion differed from theirs, I don't think that she ever sort of won that battle, basically they just demanded that they get their way . . .

. . . pretty much whatever was written on the chart or whatever they [the midwives] had been told [by the paediatricians] they just sort of did, there wasn't really a lot of worrying about what you really thought about it . . . we weren't really keen on the blood glucose tests . . . but I'm not sure if we really objected to them doing them over and over again how difficult it would have been to get that through to them at all, because they didn't really seem willing to sort of bend on that issue, they were very firm that they needed to do this and had to do it every so often . . . '

Service scenario 6

Community midwives commonly work in both community and hospital settings.

Community midwife(2)

'I think there's less preconception about what each others' roles [midwives and social workers] are than compared to say with a GP and a midwife . . . I think the social workers know where we're coming from, know what we've got to do and then they'll say their bit . . . the roles are much more defined in a sense because there hasn't been that connection historically; whereas with a GP and a midwife that's evolved . . . the GP felt that the midwife belonged to their surgery, whereas I don't think there's ever been that kind of thing . . . the two professions [midwifery and social work] are very separate . . . a midwife and a social worker . . . in some ways more equal . . . they're not coming from a medical model and they're funded in a completely different way . . . when I've had dealings with social workers it's been very much a kind of mutual respect for each other's profession but they're quite distinct.

. . . again historically [health visitors] were nurses, midwives and then health visitors, and so you've got that hierarchy in place . . . I went to a study day with a lot of health visitors . . . the midwives were outnumbered by the health visitors and I really remember feeling a little bit condescended to . . . I could see that it was grounded much more in, "Oh, I used to be a midwife and now I'm a health visitor" . . . there's definitely a potential for antagonism between the midwife and the health visitor, because we hand over to the health visitor . . . kind of rivalry there . . . I don't know why that is, it's very strange, I suppose because they're coming from a more health-policing role . . . it's all very much about social control; whereas I think midwives – although there are elements of that in the way that we screen things, screen and weigh and promote various things – I think midwives are a little bit more of a law unto themselves and I don't know why that is, I've thought about it an awful lot and I still can't come up with an answer but there's a little bit more, rebellion in midwives, I think . . . I think health visitors generally tend to be a bit more by the book, but . . . that's just an incredible overview, I mean you know I've met health visitors that aren't like that at all and you know, I've definitely met some that are scary.'

Community midwife(3)

'The paediatricians are very more . . . they're very hot on doing lots of observations and things on babies, and weighing babies, and doing all these things which I just wasn't used to when I came here [to the unit] . . . we did the minimum really with babies . . . we didn't even take their temperatures, really, and I think they're a lot more hot here on actually doing temperatures and doing things like that, as opposed to leaving us to look at a baby and say, "This is a well baby", "This isn't a well baby" . . . I hate it. I think it's horrible . . . I was talking to someone else who I trained with a while ago, and I said I think my observation skills of babies are not the same, not as good, because I'm relying on taking temperatures and doing things like that, as opposed to stripping off a baby, maybe, and just looking at it, and feeling it.

. . . some of the babies that they class as small for dates, as well, the paediatricians can be quite funny about them and they say, "Oh, they've got to have two weight gains before they go home", and you say, " Well actually, they're feeding really well, they're weeing, they're pooing, they're pink and warm . . . the weight was only this", and you have to sort of be a bit forceful with them sometimes . . . it tends to be at the SHO level, rather than above, and if you get past the SHOs, the registrars will be thoroughly sensible about things and listen to what you say . . . I don't know, whether because they're sort of fairly inexperienced and they're going by the letter of the guidelines, whereas with the registrars you can sort of say, "Well, look, it's doing all these things it should be doing, yes it hasn't had a weight gain, but it's not unwell in any way."'

Summary

Chapter 2 provided opportunities to consider the influence of senior medical staff on interprofessional working in acute care. This chapter provides further opportunities to consider interprofessional working amongst doctors and allied professionals, notably midwives. It also offers an opportunity to reflect on the role of senior midwives in supporting effective interprofessional working between two professions and amongst all grades of staff.

REFLECTIVE ACTIVITY

From the accounts presented here, what are your views on the key relationships that ensure effective care?

The accounts of women receiving maternity services, however, suggest that despite professionals' positive assessments of interprofessional working, women are highly critical of professional and interprofessional communication. Services are not presented as user-centred and providing individualized care remains a considerable challenge. The voices provide examples of how women can experience the service as being medically dominated. The accounts towards the end of the chapter suggest that there is a lack of consensus across professional groups and there are hints of concerns about professional status that can inhibit development of trust. In this specialized area of practice, consider what supports and inhibits good interprofessional working for the benefit of the service user. Reflect on your observations and consider if the factors you have identified are relevant across all settings, or whether some factors are specific to maternity care.

Review your observations after you have read each chapter in Part II.

Notes

1 DH (1993) *Changing Childbirth: Report of the Expert Maternity Group*. London:HMSO.
2 European Foundation for the Improvement of Living and Working Conditions (2004) www.eiro.eurofound.eu.int/2004/04/feature/uk0404105f.html (Accessed 01.05.2008).

References

DH (1998) *Vitamin K for Newborn Babies*. London:Department of Health.
NMC (2004) *Nursing and Midwifery Council [Midwives] Rules 2004*. London:Nursing and Midwifery Council.
Pollard K (2007) *Discourses of unity and division: a study of interprofessional working among midwives in an English NHS maternity unit*. PhD thesis, University of the West of England, Bristol.
Silverton L (1993) *The Art and Science of Midwifery*. Hemel Hempstead:Prentice Hall.

Mental Health Care

Material collated by
Paul Godin and Margaret Miers

This chapter draws on data from three research studies. Interviews with mental health students and with qualified staff during a longitudinal evaluation of a pre-qualifying interprofessional curriculum provide perspectives from community and care of older people settings (Pollard *et al.* 2007, 2008). Perspectives from forensic mental health are drawn from a three-year qualitative study of a forensic mental health unit (Davies *et al.* 2006, Godin *et al.* 2006, Shaw *et al.* 2007) and a pilot project on user involvement in research (Godin *et al.* 2007).

Student perspectives

Mental health nursing students, interviewed about their experiences of interprofessional working in placement settings, were able to comment on working patterns that inhibited or supported interprofessional collaboration and on the complexity of collaborative working skills.

Mental health nursing student(1)

'This placement in particular has given me a lot of insight into how not to function as a professional because we have here, we have separate teams. We have three CPN [Community Psychiatric Nurse] teams, we have an OT [Occupational Therapy] team which is separate from the CPNs and we have a social work team who is separate . . . and it's pants. People don't stay here for very long. I can see why they don't stay here long: because there is no working together. Workloads are horrendous. OTs have their meetings in the morning, social workers have their meetings in the morning and the CPNs have their meetings in the morning. So information isn't passed on. Communication is really quite poor. And yet everyone is stressing because their workload is so high and this, that and the other. And yet if people actually sat down and spoke to each other it would be a lot easier. If they were all together it would be helpful.'

Mental health nursing student(2): older people assessment centre

'One thing that struck me about the ward rounds was the consultant was kind of chairing the meeting as well as having to make potentially life-, you know, not life-threatening, but life-saving decisions about medication; and the first one that I went to she was very professional, but I felt as if, by the end of the hour – it was hot, the sun was coming into the room, she was struggling somewhat because she was controlling . . . I don't know why she was controlling, but she was controlling the course of the meeting and she had to prompt everyone, everyone's opinions about each service user and go through one to the other, and it was taking that all on board. I felt that maybe the ward manager should have chaired the meeting and given the consultant a chance to digest the information. 'Cos that's something that came out in our IP [interprofessional] module as well.'

'And do you think that the consultant felt she just had to do it because of her role?'

'Well, possibly. 'Cos that's something that I read about in the literature on it. But there's, I think it would only add to the "doctor knows best" culture and doctors are more intelligent than other professionals below, but they are only human at the end of the day. If they have travelled all that way they might be very good at rationally thinking things through in terms of medicine, but dealing with a whole group of people and thinking about medical matters at the same time, I think is inefficient.'

Qualified staff perspectives

In the interprofessional curriculum evaluation qualified practitioners were interviewed about their experience of interprofessional learning and interprofessional working. Qualified staff described examples of interprofessional working that were particularly memorable, either because the experience of interprofessional collaboration had led to a positive outcome for service users, or because failures in collaborative working had contributed to negative experiences.

Social worker(3): adult community care

'When you undertake an assessment it's usually allocated to a specific person but there's usually two people that go out to complete the assessment . . . and I can think of one occasion when I went out with a consultant psychiatrist . . .

and you could view that as a bit of a luxury really . . . we had the referral come through . . . It was asking for respite care . . . and this is why the referral forms need to be comprehensive . . . when we went out I said to him before we went into the house, "Can I ask you why you would have this referral? What's the consultant psychiatrist's role in this? It's primarily respite; why would you be involved?" He said, "To be honest I don't know why I've been asked to come along, what my role is going to be. But let's go in . . . keep an open mind . . . we'll go in together." We spoke to the carer and she was really, really stressed . . . about the behavioural difficulties her husband was exhibiting . . . Now if I had been a lone worker . . . as we are in the disabled adults team . . . I would go out and you would recognize the difficulties. But you wouldn't necessarily pick up on what the consultant psychiatrist picked up on, which was the medication. [The husband] had been prescribed medication that had interacted with other medications that he was prescribed and that was causing him to exhibit some of the behaviour that he was exhibiting. What actually happened as a consequence of that . . . he was admitted to the ward for assessment. They looked at the whole picture . . . did a whole medication review to wean him off the medication in a supervised setting. Now if I'd gone out on my own I wouldn't necessarily have been aware of this . . . and we could have masked the problem.'

Social worker(4): care management team

'We had a case recently where there was an older woman . . . and there were lots of concerns that police were coming to us and that and when we went there she wouldn't let us in . . . and eventually we got the [area] service involved, which is the mental health [service] in this area. Now I'd gone out there with another colleague because we were worried about this person and the police were and we then passed it over to our other colleagues' service . . . to say that we wanted a mental health assessment . . . and she agreed to that. Now I presumed that was going on and a whole week later I had an email to say that this woman was found dead in her flat. Now the repercussions and how that made me feel and my anger and I don't often get angry and I was really . . . upset that the system had failed her and that I'd been naïve enough to presume that it was going on, so it was a learning curve for me . . . and there was an investigation and some of that came down to workload, but it left me really, really upset on that one because we'd failed the service user completely . . . and how our colleagues the police view us now, I should not think in a very good light . . .

. . . Some of that came down to, letting each other know . . . if only they'd phoned me and left a message and emailed me to say we've changed our mind, we're doing this . . . we're going to send somebody else in . . . we've not got in . . .

. . . and you've got to work through then how you feel towards your other professionals, which I found very hard for a few weeks . . . That was just an extreme example of what happened and lack of communication . . . we failed her. And some of that came down to communication . . .

. . . the police . . . the weekend she died, had actually been called out again and she turned down going away, so that's why I say the outcome would have been the same, no matter what, but it was just that as professionals somebody hadn't respected me enough to let me know they hadn't gone out, and me as a professional should have checked it out as well, not just left it, so there's a lot of learning curves on that, but that was not very good interprofessional working at all . . . I don't know whether if they'd known me more they would have respected my professionalism more, and my concerns more if they'd known me, I don't know . . . and it really is talking to one another, isn't it? How many times do you hear that? It's the same lack of talking to one another isn't it?'

Mental health nurse(1): eating disorders unit

'My current post is Day Therapy Co-ordinator. The day-therapy programme is for people with eating disorders. On a day-to-day basis I work with dieticians, occupational therapists, physiotherapists, art psychotherapists, clinical psychologists, psychiatrists. We ask those attending the programme to do a range of tasks: some of them basically general tasks around rehabilitating their eating; others are therapeutic tasks. I co-ordinate this programme so I make sure that all those kind of things happen, and that requires interaction with my colleagues from various disciplines in terms of making things happen but also in terms of ensuring progression . . . monitoring and assessing progress . . . so I kind of work with people on a range of levels . . .

. . . I think one of the issues about the programme – and this was organized before I was involved with the team – is that for everybody, those kind of professional boundaries and differences are very much flattened and blurred, so although there are people here with years and years of experience and lots of qualifications and are much higher on the banding, for instance, than I am . . . we pretty much operate and treat each other as equal.'

'Overall, then, how would you rate the interprofessional collaboration in your workplace?'

'I think it's excellent. You know, I don't know of any other unit . . . in eating disorders or not that operates in this way and I think it's highly beneficial . . . it's a great benefit to team, team coherence really. I think it delivers care in a much more effective way . . .

. . . I think it's the communication and being able to sit down with one another and discuss things, and although we do recognize boundaries and certain strengths . . . at certain points I think we come together around them rather than fall apart because of them and we as a team have a regular supervision and discuss things regularly, so I think we're managed really, really well and this all adds up to being very, very helpful.'

'Right. And so do you get the opportunity to have regular sort of team meetings?'

'We have team meetings every week and we have a team supervision for the team every month and we also have supervision every month at least around the Day Therapy programme as well . . . so we're fortunate in that sense that we have a lot of time, and we make sure we make a lot of space to be able to do those things.'

'How would you say that the interprofessional working impacts on the actual service delivery?'

'I think the service delivery is more coherent, especially in this area of mental health where people generally have a range of needs, both mental and physical. I think to have these crossovers is very, very important and so we can provide a really full service and a broad service and I think people really, really benefit from that. There's a range of professions, there's a whole range of personalities, which really helps the mix and helps . . . they are quite a diverse range of people we see, so it's been nothing but a positive experience for me . . .

. . . I think other teams in eating disorders particularly find a very strong division of tasks . . . kind of the nurses and the OTs do all the food-based stuff and the psychologists and psychiatrists do all the mind-based stuff. That has been . . . dissolved almost . . . and I think . . . everybody is involved and everybody can play a part . . . and is seen as very important, which I think is really, really useful. So I think the way of working as a whole by the team has been led by the team leader here has been very, very important to me.'

'Thinking more generally about interprofessional working, what sorts of skills or abilities or qualities do you think that professionals need in order to work effectively as members of interprofessional teams?'

'I think you need to have a knowledge of what other people do . . . there are lots of opportunities for certain myths to build up about what people do and do not do and what are their tasks and what are their responsibilities. Understanding people's skill bases is really, really important and it helps to inform your own practice and skills but also in terms of trying to think about appropriate interventions for a client . . .

. . . I also think there's a certain amount of cross-pollination of skills and knowledge . . . you're just exposed to, I guess, different ideas, different philosophies, different practices, different ways of working which again can inform your own practice and help shape your own practice. I'm very much of a point of view of mongrels last longer than pedigree dogs . . . I'm very happy to sort of pick and mix skills and . . . this here right now feels a very rich environment for that . . . for instance I trained in a particular therapy . . . last year and the majority . . . on the course were psychologists but it was no issue to go from this team and do that . . .

. . . it's very important for what we deliver that it is a multidisciplinary, multiprofessional way of working because in terms of thinking about eating disorders, there is no one way that works . . . psychologists or psychiatrists don't have the magic answer . . . you have to think all across the board and that's why we need people to bring all of their skills to what we do.'

Forensic mental health care unit

In a three-year qualitative study of a forensic unit (Davies *et al.* 2006, Godin *et al.* 2006, Shaw *et al.* 2007), data were collected through observations, field visits, interviews, patient-centred case studies and staff seminars (including a multidisciplinary team workshop). The unit accommodated almost 100 patients, who were looked after by approximately 300 professionals, comprising nurses, doctors, managers, occupational therapists, psychologists, social therapists and social workers. Additionally, the unit also employed a substantial number of cleaners, receptionists, administrators and other support staff.

Different systems

Being in and between the health and penal systems clearly gave rise to differences in opinion amongst the staff as to whether their role was to do with custody or care.

Nurse manager

'There's always what I call a battle between the hawks and the doves. The hawks will shut everything down and become the Prisoner Officers' Association. They would tend to be over the top and real authoritarian. They don't see patients as individuals, they see them as prisoners. The doves want to liberate, they're very much in a therapeutic community mode which I've got a lot of sympathy for, I've worked in one before. But at the same time, they are so loose and so liberal that they've lost the plot and they really need to be aware that this is a regional secure unit and a real exercise for security and that's about people owning that and owning that responsibility and I think at times that gets lost with some of the staff here.'

Risk perception

Whilst service users had been placed in the unit because of the risk they putatively posed, health care professionals were employed to deal with that risk. Although service users and the various professional groups that cared for them all shared the task of having to address this risk, they all understood and dealt with it very differently. Whereas service users commonly denied or minimized being a threat, each of the professions conceptualized and managed the risk that patients posed from their different disciplinary perspectives. As a psychologist politely explained, psychiatrists' risk assessments centre around the identification and treatment of mental disorders whilst psychological assessments go beyond such considerations.

Psychologist

'It might be not entirely accurate to say that psychiatry is mostly looking at mental disorder but, but I mean they work within a medical framework so they, they're making a diagnosis of mental disorder, you know, they're pre-scribing treatments. Of course they have an interest in risk, and I, I suppose my experience of working in a multidisciplinary team is that that is debated really, but that you know, I would see the psychological assessment as being quite a key one really, because, well, I think everybody would agree that risk isn't just to do with a mental disorder, you know, you have to look at a lot of other things as well.'

Risk and unit structure

Within the highly regulated and hierarchically ordered structure of the unit, service users and each of the professional groups additionally faced very differ-ent risks associated with the particular roles they were each obliged to play. Service users feared the risks of becoming institutionalized and being mis-treated. Nurses bore a major responsibility for operating a bureaucratic system for the maintenance of security within the unit. In so doing they faced the risk of being blamed for breaches in security when patients escaped, harmed others or themselves. Meanwhile, as leaders, managers and consultant psychiatrists were responsible for the unit's overall success, indicated by such outcomes as good interprofessional working, and thus ran the risk of being discredited as ineffectual.

The thinking and associated actions of service users and health care profes-sions were also strongly influenced by their alliances. In individual interviews, members of each occupational group loyally expressed their own tribe's ideo-logical view of what caused the service users' problems, drawing attention to the uniquely special contribution their own professional group made in care, treatment and risk management.

Interprofessional collaboration

Observational data proved particularly telling in understanding which ideas and values expressed by staff and patients were actually translated into action Although nurses and non-medical staff voiced objections in interviews to the limitations of the medical perspective and medical dominance, they did not always express these views in forums for interprofessional discussion, such as ward rounds and case conferences.

The general view of staff within the unit was that interprofessional working was a desirable ideal that was only ever partially realized. Participants viewed interprofessional work very differently according to their position within the hierarchical regulation of the unit. Whereas in individual interviews nurses commonly blamed psychiatrists' domineering approach and assertion of the medical model for failure in interprofessional working, the problem was seen differently from the psychiatrists' perspective.

Psychiatrist

'Here, I am happy, the team here is very supportive, a very supportive team, yes, I suppose a multi-, well it is difficult, there's a multidisciplinary split as well, there is a split in my view between the nursing staff and everybody else and it has been extremely difficult to get the nursing staff to share the vision in the same way as the rest of the multidisciplinary team . . . '

Nursing perspectives

Whilst shadowing another consultant on his morning of ward-round meetings one of the researchers noticed how the nursing staff were sometimes reluctant to join the meeting. On one ward an agency nurse eventually arrived at the meeting to report on the progress of a patient he did not even know. Although the consultant regarded this behaviour as indicative of nurses' indifference to interprofessional practice, a different explanation emerged at a subsequent multidisciplinary workshop organized by the research team. Despite their putative lack of interest in interprofessional working, 14 nurses attended, along with four health care assistants, three occupational therapists and one administrator. Although a consultant psychiatrist had registered for the workshop, there were no psychiatrists actually present, neither were there any social workers or psychologists. As nurses dominated the workshop it was not surprising that they began rehearsing their complaint that interprofessional working was stifled by medical domination. As discussion progressed to the topic of risk assessment and risk management, an occupational therapist made the following interesting observation.

Occupational therapist(2)

'There is something I noticed in the low secure ward . . . It was sort of set up to be more multidisciplinary. But, since then, there has been a rain [cluster] of incidents. And, because of the blame culture, the discipline [nursing] is increasingly retreating into themselves. You know, the nurses start being particularly blamed and . . . it's extremely difficult for them to sort of maintain their prominence and significance in the multidisciplinary team . . . There is a fear of actually engaging in the multidisciplinary process because that is a potential for further blame' (Shaw *et al.* 2007:369).

Blame

Perhaps nurses' reluctance to participate in ward rounds and other interprofessional forums was less to do with apathy and indifference and more to do with retreating from a situation in which blame was loaded upon them. This perceived tendency to blame nurses for the failings of the unit was also expressed in individual interviews.

The blaming of nurses caused them to recoil from interprofessional discussion forums, silencing nurses' opposition to what they perceived to be the inadequacies of the medical model, whilst bolstering medical domination.

Manager

''cos nursing here is traditional, when there's been a cock-up or a mistake they're [nurses] the ones that bend down and touch their toes and all other professionals come along and give them a good kick' (Godin *et al.* 2006: 85).

Nursing officer

'I think too often in past here the nurses have just gone along and they've been mute. There is a medical model here . . . there's one or two [consultant psychiatrists] who are very much the old school, you know, "I snap my fingers and you as a nurse do what I say" . . . '

Service users

Though the term interprofessional or multidisciplinary working is generally regarded as virtuous and was unopposed as a desirable ideal by the staff of the unit, the term implicitly suggests that service users do not have a real part to play in its collaborative procedure. Their only contribution is as consumers who might give their opinion about the services professionals provide, which regulate patients' behaviour within a secure (prison-like) environment.

In a separate, forensic service user-led research study (Godin *et al.* 2007), it became very apparent that service users often fear and second-guess what records are being constructed and what is being said about them in ward rounds, case conferences and handovers. Furthermore, forensic service users often felt that the staff 'stuck together' whenever patients complained about the service provided and constructed untruths about patients to discredit their testimonies. Although, as we have seen, professionals felt interprofessional work was not always effective, the service users saw the staff as very united in their practice, albeit in a rather negative way. However, their view of interprofessional working was not always so jaundiced. Service users also identified times when professionals had worked sensitively and collaboratively to facilitate something they enjoyed, as the following story illustrates.

Service user(5)

'My social worker, she had a . . . labrador, she used to bring him for walks . . . I was allowed to walk the dog around the grounds. I'd be there all afternoon. It is so relaxing, I come back on the ward after, and I was so relaxed and cheerful and happy, that the doctor asked [social worker] to bring the dog in every week . . . pet therapy. And it really does work. And that is what we did each week.'

Summary

The views of students and qualified staff reported in the first half of this chapter have been informed by their own experiences of interprofessional education. A focus on interprofessional learning and working in their pre-qualifying curriculum may have alerted them to the importance of skills, attitudes and organizational factors in supporting positive interprofessional working relationships. The mental health nurse working in a unit for people with eating disorders reports excellent interprofessional relationships but, in contrast, voices from the forensic mental health unit present a picture of a hierarchically structured unit in which separate professions were perceived as working as separate tribes. Throughout the chapter different voices identify the importance of demonstrating respect for other professionals and the damaging consequences for service users and for professionals themselves when such respect breaks down.

REFLECTIVE ACTIVITY

Make a note of the key points that emerge for you from the accounts in this chapter. Reflect on the difference between positive and negative examples of interprofessional teamwork in mental health care and consider strategies for improving interprofessional working in the forensic mental health unit. Could interprofessional education make a difference and if so, how?

Review your reflections after you have read each chapter in Part II.

References

Davies J, Heyman B, Godin P, Shaw M, Reynolds L (2006) The problems of offenders with mental disorders: a plurality of perspectives within a single mental health care organization. *Social Science & Medicine* 63:1097–108.

Godin P, Davies J, Heyman B, Reynolds L, Simpson A, Floyd M (2007) Open communicative space: a Habermasian understanding of a user-led participatory research project. *Journal of Forensic Psychiatry and Psychology* 18(4):452–69.

Godin P, Davies J, Heyman B, Shaw M (2006) Different understandings of risk within a forensic mental health care unit: a cultural approach. In: Godin P (ed) *Risk and Nursing Practice*. Basingstoke:Palgrave Macmillan, 79–97.

Pollard K, Rickaby C, Miers M (2008) *Evaluating Student Learning in an Interprofessional Curriculum: The Relevance of Pre-qualifying Interprofessional Education for Future Professional Practice*. HEA Health Science and Practice Subject Centre with UWE, Bristol. www.health. heacademy.ac.uk/projects/miniprojects/completeproj.htm (Accessed 7.12.08).

Pollard K, Rickaby C, Ventura S, Ross K, Taylor P, Evans D, Harrison J (2007) *Transference to Practice (TOP): A Study of Collaborative Learning and Working in Placement Settings. The Student Voice*. Bristol:University of the West of England. http://hsc.uwe.ac.uk/net/research/ Default.aspx?pageid=29 (Accessed 7.12.08).

Shaw M, Heyman B, Reynolds L, Davies J, Godin P (2007) Multidisciplinary teamwork in a UK regional secure mental health unit a matter for negotiation? *Social Theory and Health* 5:356–77.

PART II

Analysing the Issues

Introduction
Katherine C Pollard

We hope, as editors, that readers will by now have had the opportunity to familiarize themselves with the material in Part I; and with the aid of the reflective activities at the end of each chapter, will have started to consider some of the issues influencing and raised by interprofessional working in the contexts and environments described by the different 'voices'. The presentation of various theoretical perspectives in Part II is designed to assist readers in extending their knowledge and developing their ways of thinking about some of these issues, and about the complex process that constitutes interprofessional working in health and social care in a modern Western society.

Chapter authors were asked to write about a particular theoretical area, and were provided with the material in Part I in order to illustrate their discussion. The authors have included further activities for readers in each chapter, in order to encourage engagement with relevant issues.

In Chapter 6, Margaret Miers considers theories explaining how individuals learn to operate in multiprofessional settings, as well as identifying and discussing relevant factors that influence learning in practice. Diverse literature exploring learning, professional socialization and professional knowledge and practice shares an interest in the situated nature of learning. A range of learning theories are discussed in this context, including Piaget's (1958) theories of cognitive development, as well as social learning theories such as Wenger's (1998) 'communities of practice' and Engeström's (2001) work on activity theory. Attention is also paid to issues concerning support for learning, development of appropriate skills and the merits of interprofessional education.

Billie Oliver and Celia Keeping address issues of individual and professional identity in Chapter 7. The focus of the chapter is the construction of 'occupational identity' rather than the factors contributing to an individual's status as 'a professional'. The authors accordingly explore questions such as: What does calling oneself a 'social worker' or a 'nurse' mean in identity terms? And what happens to that sense of identity when the boundary between 'nurse' and 'social worker' becomes blurred through new integrated practices? The chapter includes consideration of the agency/structure dichotomy and the relationship between identity and structural influences, while drawing on theories of personal and social identity to help understand experiences of interprofessional working. Key approaches explored include those linking individual agency with identity, such as Erikson's (1968) 'life-span theory' of identity development, social identity theory (Stets and Burke 2000) and community identity (Adams and Marshall 1996). The authors also consider late modern and postmodern approaches to understanding identities as shifting, fragmented and incomplete rather than stable and unified, including the idea of 'challenged identities' (Ibarra 2003), and apply this understanding to the complexity that interprofessional working introduces.

In Chapter 8, Margaret Miers addresses concerns about professional boundaries, which can inhibit the effectiveness of interprofessional working. This is a significant issue, as modernizing health and social care services involves a constant shifting of professional activities and boundaries. This chapter explores approaches to understanding professions, professionalization and the relationship between professions and the state as well as the relationship between professional development and changing technologies. A range of theories is considered, including those which have stressed the competitive and exclusionary aspects of professionalism (Freidson 1970), those arguing for a 'new model' of professionalism (Davies 1995), and those exploring demarcatory strategies as practices of occupational closure, deriving from professional conflict (Witz 1992). Negotiation around professional boundaries in interprofessional working is discussed with particular reference to the work of Nancarrow and Borthwick (2005), who have described four types of boundary change: diversification, specialization, horizontal substitution and vertical substitution.

In Chapter 9, Katherine C Pollard revisits the medicalization thesis in the current social context, which includes the feminization of the workplace and the rise of the discourse of the marketplace in health and social care services (Nye 2003, Nettleton 2006). Cultural aspects of interprofessional interaction are examined, as exemplified in the case-study material, in relation to the medicalization thesis. Factors discussed include medical dominance, with reference to the privileging of medical knowledge and the medical perspective within the wider social context, as well as within health and social care organizations and structures. How status deriving from medical dominance affects interprofessional relationships, including those which involve non-professional staff and service users, is also considered. Discussion of the nature of hierarchies, teams and leadership is included. The author explores the possibilities for parity within interprofessional relationships in health and social care in a society that privileges the medical viewpoint and endorses the medicalization of a range of social issues. Ongoing tensions between health care and social care are addressed with reference to the medicalization thesis. The complex interaction between medical dominance and issues of gender and power are discussed in relation to wider social factors.

In Chapter 10, Tim Harle and his co-authors apply organizational theory to interprofessional working. The current emphasis on interprofessional working can be viewed in the context of new organizational forms and approaches to management and leadership that emphasize flat rather than hierarchical structures. In addition, workforce change in health and social care reflects wider changes in labour markets and patterns of work organization. This chapter brings two particular perspectives to bear: first, that of developments in the field of leadership within organizations, citing, among others, the work of Schein (2004); secondly, that of complexity theory (Wheatley 2005, Sarra 2006), in which new theories about the ways that organizations function are applied to the interprofessional context within health and social care. Throughout the chapter, the authors maintain an emphasis on the necessity to maintain awareness of service user needs when addressing organizational and system issues in interprofessional working.

In Chapter 11, Derek Sellman focuses on values and ethics in relation to interprofessional working. On the face of it, there would seem to be more that unites than divides the values guiding health and social care practice. This is because the primary purpose of health and social care practice is human betterment and, as such, serves as a core value for the 'helping' professions (which include health and social care professions). Working towards human betterment involves adhering to a basic set of commitments that places prohibitions, for example, on killing patients or on intentionally inflicting unnecessary harm. While these may come with caveats, the general thrust of the prohibitions is fundamental to health or social care practice, and this goes some way to explain the rather attractive idea of a common value base for all health and social care professionals. However, differences in values and priorities between specific professions can have a detrimental effect on interprofessional relationships in health and social care. Following a discussion of act-based and agent-based ethics (Hursthouse 1997, Beauchamp and Childress 2001), the author identifies and explores three conditions related to ethics and values which he considers necessary for effective interprofessional practice: willingness, trust and leadership.

In Chapter 12, Judith Thomas considers the position of service users and carers.

This chapter explores user and carer involvement in the development of services at different levels. It draws on the perspectives of users and carers in relation to interprofessional issues and examines associated benefits, tensions and dilemmas. The author draws on theories of power and empowerment (Foucault 2000, Faulkner 2001, Payne 2002) to consider how collaborative practice can be enhanced and theoretical frameworks developed. Particular attention is paid to terminology, information giving, 'ownership' of service users and the development of service user power and control.

As can be seen from the above, Part II comprises an eclectic range of theory. However, owing to space and other constraints, consideration of the effects of pertinent cultural, ethnic and religious factors on interprofessional working have not been included. Nevertheless, the editors have aimed to present a variety of theories: those which address particular professional issues, as well as those which apply to wider societal perspectives.

Making the most of Part II

The activities included in each chapter afford readers the opportunity to engage more closely with the phenomenon of interprofessional working, as conceptualized through the lens of a particular theory. Through this engagement with the range of theoretical perspectives provided, and with reference to the 'voices' in Part I, it is anticipated that, despite inevitable omissions, readers will be able to explore new ways of framing ideas about interprofessional working through which they may extend their understanding of relevant issues in their professional practice.

References

Adams GR, Marshall SK (1996) A developmental social psychology of identity: understanding the person-in-context. *Journal of Adolescence* 19:429–42.

Beauchamp T, Childress T (2001) *Principles of Biomedical Ethics.* (5th edn) Oxford:Oxford University Press.

Davies C (1995) *Gender and the Professional Predicament in Nursing.* Buckingham:Open University Press.

Engeström Y (2001) Expansive learning at work: toward an activity theoretical reconceptualisation. *Journal of Education and Work* 14(1):133–56.

Erikson EH (1968) *Identity: Youth and Crisis.* New York:Norton.

Faulkner M (2001) Models of empowerment and disempowerment. *NT research* 6(6):936–48.

Foucault M (2000) *Power.* Ed JD Faubion. New York:The New Press.

Freidson E (1970) *Profession of Medicine: A Study of the Sociology of Applied Knowledge.* Chicago:University of Chicago Press.

Hursthouse R (1997) Virtue ethics and abortion. In: Statman D (ed) *Virtue Ethics: A Critical Reader.* Edinburgh:Edinburgh University Press, 227–44.

Ibarra H (2003) *Working Identity: Unconventional Strategies for Reinventing Your Career.* Boston:Harvard Business School Press.

Nancarrow SA, Borthwick AM (2005) Dynamic professional boundaries in the health care workforce. *Sociology of Health and Illness* 27(7):897–919.

Nettleton S (2006) *The Sociology of Health and Illness.* (2nd edn) Cambridge:Polity Press.

Nye R (2003) The evolution of the concept of medicalization in the late twentieth century. *Journal of History of the Behavioural Sciences* 39(2):115–29.

Payne M (2002) The role and achievements of a professional association in the later twentieth century: the British association of social workers 1970–2000. *British Journal of Social Work* 32(8):969–95.

Piaget J (1958) *The Growth of Logical Thinking from Childhood to Adolescence.* New York:Basic Books.

Sarra N (2006) *The Emotional Experience of Performance Management in the Health Sector: The Corridor.* In: Stacey R, Griffin D (eds) *Complexity and the Experience of Managing in the Public Sector.* London:Routledge, 81–107.

Schein E (2004) *Organizational Culture and Leadership.* (3rd edn) San Francisco:Jossey-Bass.

Stets JE, Burke PJ (2000) Identity theory and social identity theory. *Social Psychology Quarterly* 63(3):224–37.

Wenger E (1998) *Communities of Practice: Learning, Meaning and Identity.* Cambridge:Cambridge University Press.

Wheatley M (2005) *Finding Our Way.* San Francisco:Berrett-Koehler.

Witz A (1992) *Professions and Patriarchy.* London:Routledge.

CHAPTER

6

Learning for New Ways of Working

Margaret Miers

Introduction

Health and social care have not always been provided by professionals. In the pre-industrial era such care was mainly provided by women within the family and the local community. The development of knowledge-based occupations was a slow process, partly dependent on the development of training schools, and, for medicine and law, access to university-based education. In Britain, for example, the Medical Registration Act was passed in 1858 (Witz 1992), requiring medical practitioners to pass examinations before practising. A Nurse Registration Bill was passed in 1919 (Dingwall *et al.* 1988, Miers 2000), the Chartered Society of Physiotherapy was established in 1944, evolving from the Society of Trained Masseurs established in 1894 (Hawes and Rees 2005), and the first occupational therapy training school (Dorset House in Bristol) opened in the UK in 1930 (Wilcock 2002). The history of many health professions is a history of progressive attainment of professional autonomy over their own area of practice, control over their own education, and regulation by professional bodies and councils established by the government, for example the General Medical Council (GMC), the Nursing and Midwifery Council (NMC), the Health Professions Council (HPC) and the General Social Care Council (GSCC), which take responsibility for the registers of practitioners. The HPC is responsible for 13 separate professions, all claiming distinctive expertise (see Barrett *et al.* 2005, Health Professions Council www.hpc-uk.org/). The importance of specialist skills and knowledge was recognized by the movement of nursing and allied health professions' education into universities in the

1990s. However, this movement towards graduate status can be seen as exacerbating the emphasis on the difference between professions. To date, only nursing remains a non-graduate profession. The NMC has, however, declared the intention to move towards graduate status (NMC 2008).

It is hardly surprising that this expansion in independent health and social care professions has led to concern about the negative impact of separate professional cultures developing through professional socialization. Gaining state recognition for professional status has often been a conflictual process, with occupational groups both expanding and protecting their areas of practice, as Chapter 8 explores. Separate professional preparation programmes have led to each profession having a different 'cognitive map' (Petrie 1976), which can inhibit shared understanding of a problem. Hall (2005:191) argues that largely unspoken and implicit professional value systems 'can create important obstacles that may actually be invisible to different team members struggling with a problem'. The negative impact of professional silos on the delivery of care has been internationally recognized. In the UK, the Department of Health, in *The NHS Plan* (DH 2000), suggested the development of a common foundation programme for health professionals to increase professionals' understanding of each other, aid co-operation and support career and workforce flexibility. Confusion about the nature, content and purpose of such a programme, however, has meant that UK higher education institutions have not pursued this idea. In contrast, providing opportunities for students to learn together in interprofessional groups has been commonplace. Interprofessional learning – learning from, with and about each other (CAIPE 1997) – is seen as a mechanism for supporting effective interprofessional collaboration and reducing barriers to teamwork created by separate educational programmes.

It is the voluntary sector workers in Chapter 3 who show most awareness of the negative impact of 'silo' professional education. The manager of a large voluntary agency (MLVA) notes the difficulties of developing a participation strategy for children and their families and carers because

> different professional groups have very different understanding, experiences and attitudes around participation and there can be tensions around this.

The community development worker expresses scepticism about the narrowness of professional expertise:

> I make a point of not minding to ask stupid questions . . . I find myself piping up a lot and saying, 'What does that mean?' and it'll turn out that quite a lot of other people in the room won't know what it means either; because they're coming from different disciplines.

In order to support collaboration around the Sure Start initiative, the MLVA described training opportunities designed to share information about professional roles.

We had a system where at inter-agency team meetings, people took it in turns to talk about their roles and it was open to anyone working or funded by Sure Start to participate. Different professions would take the agenda for half an hour and share what they thought others needed to know about their service and interprofessional and inter-agency dilemmas and issues.

The account of interprofessional working in a forensic mental health unit in Chapter 5 illustrates the difficulties separate professional cultures can create. In such a setting there are differences in opinion about whether professional roles involve custody or care and differences in opinion about the relevance of a medical framework in determining treatment. A nurse manager spoke about 'a battle between the hawks and the doves':

> The hawks will shut everything down and become the Prisoner Officers' Association . . . they don't see patients as individuals, they see them as prisoners. The doves want to liberate, they're very much in a therapeutic community mode.

A psychologist perceived differences between assessment of risk by psychiatrists and clinical psychologists, with psychiatrists focusing on the diagnosis and treatment of mental disorders and psychologists looking 'at a lot of other things as well'.

Professional socialization

Professional education is not just a process of gaining knowledge and skills, it is a process of socialization into the values and characteristics of a professional group. Goodwin (1994:606) writes about the development of 'professional vision' as 'socially organised ways of seeing and understanding events that are answerable to the distinctive interests of a particular social group'. Studies of medical socialization have explored processes whereby medical students learn the practices of senior physicians in order to manage the uncertainties that characterize professional work (Fox 1975[1957]). Haas and Saffir (1977) argued that student socialization into the medical profession involved adopting a 'cloak of competence' in order to take on the responsibility of their role. It is the importance of the need to take on medical responsibility that can lead to an emphasis on detachment and entitlement in medical training, factors which Coulehan and Williams (2001) argue can militate against more collaborative models of health care decision-making. Unsurprisingly, given the high status of doctors within the health care team, a seminal study of nurse socialization (Melia 1987) revealed that students learning to nurse learned to 'fit in' in the many different working groups they experienced during their training. Hence student nurses learned subservience both to medical dominance and to nursing's own hierarchical system.

Socialization into social work has received less attention from researchers. Barretti (2004) argues that studies of professional socialization in social work focus on the assimilation of values, thus reflecting the importance of values in social work educators' and researchers' self-perception. Nevertheless, studies have shown conflicting results, suggesting that professional education does not always lead to expected outcomes. The low status of the profession appears to create stress for social work students (Barbour 1985, Loseke and Cahill 1986). Some studies suggest that perceptions about status contribute to professional stereotypes among medical, nursing and social work students; nurses and social workers perceived medical students as superior in academic ability but lacking in breadth of experience (Carpenter 1995); social workers rated themselves positively in terms of breadth of experience but were less confident than medical students about their professional competence (Carpenter and Hewstone 1996).

ACTIVITY

If you are a member of a profession, reflect on your own professional education and think about ways in which you gained professional knowledge, skills and attitudes.

Consider the people and processes you found most influential in your professional development.

Traditional patterns of professional socialization supporting the dominance of medicine in health and social care teams are now in decline. Nevertheless, the voices in Part I illuminate the legacy of traditional hierarchies and their impact on interprofessional working. The emergency care consultant (ECC) in Chapter 2 recognizes that hierarchical systems do not work because 'people aren't empowered to speak up', but perceives that reliance on an outdated model involving the doctor thinking, 'I'm the person in charge, I'm the top of the hierarchy' persists because change is a threat to self esteem, status and position and the 'hierarchical cushion makes them feel comfortable'. The children's nurse working in acute settings describes the behaviour of the orthopaedic surgeons as characterized by 'dreadful, dreadful communication' embedded in historical and ritualistic practices.

> The orthopaedic doctors, like general surgeons, do not communicate unless they have to with anybody . . . if they can get away with speaking to a senior nurse, they won't speak to a junior nurse . . . and they don't always write in the notes . . . we have to have ESP [extra-sensory perception], or we have to go and bleep them . . . and we will say, 'Right, so you need to either come back and write in the notes or come and communicate with somebody regarding what's going on; and do we know what's going on? No, because you haven't told us, so now I'm bothering you.'

The senior registrar: paediatrics (SRP), however, demonstrates a very different approach to learning how to work in particular settings. He recognizes that hierarchical dominance can inhibit communication and is alert to the 'feel on the ward of how things are', associating relaxed conversations and informality with 'things going reasonably well'. The importance of informal learning in the workplace is now widely recognized (Eraut 1994); Pollard (2008:14) has argued that 'non-formal learning in practice settings is key to the acquisition of appropriate skills and attitudes for effective interprofessional collaboration'. In a study of student learning about interprofessional collaboration in placement settings, Pollard (2008) found that students were exposed to a wide range of practices. Whereas many students perceived interprofessional interaction to be positive, they nevertheless identified a range of suboptimal behaviour, notably lack of transfer of information, even while not necessarily recognizing it as such. Student voices in Chapter 5, however, note student awareness of their own learning in mental health settings.

> a lot of insight into how not to function as a professional because we have here, we have separate teams . . . OTs have their meetings in the morning, social workers have their meetings in the morning and the CPNs have their meetings in the morning. So information isn't passed on. Communication is really poor. And yet everyone is stressing because their workload is so high . . . if people actually sat down and spoke to each other it would be a lot easier.
>
> Mental health nursing student(1)

Mental health nursing student(2) reflected on the role of the consultant psychiatrist in a meeting:

> The consultant was kind of chairing the meeting as well as having to make potentially life-saving decisions about medication. I felt as if, by the end of the hour – it was hot . . . she was struggling somewhat because she was controlling . . . the course of the meeting and she had to prompt everyone's opinions about each service user . . . I felt that maybe the ward manager should have chaired the meeting and given the consultant a chance to digest the information.

Theories of learning

One challenge for health and social care professionals learning to work together more effectively can be a lack of shared views about how individuals learn, and particularly about learning in the workplace. Part I shows that different professions may rely on different learning approaches grounded in different theories of learning. Learning theories can be grouped together in many different ways. In the context of learning to work together one approach may be to distinguish between learning theories that focus on the individual and theories that view learning as a social process, focusing on the social environment (or workplace). Traditionally much professional education has relied on didactic models of knowledge transmission from a teacher to an individual learner, either in formal educational settings or in practice, where the learner undertakes a form of apprenticeship. Implicit in such approaches is the view that the teacher knows best, the learner receives knowledge passively, and can change behaviour after instruction. The voices in Part I suggest that didactic, teacher-led models of education have had a significant impact on medical education. In Chapter 3 the SRP comments thoughtfully on the impact of such assumptions on relationships with service users:

> I think doctors give a lot of information. I was just talking to a consultant this morning and . . . she kept describing information she was giving, she wants the patient apparently to fit in with our agenda, on the basis that if you do as we tell you, you'll get better, so if you take your treatments properly, if you have this kind of diet . . . I didn't hear a lot about, 'What are you looking for from the service?'

The language of learning adopted within the health sector can serve as a reminder of different values espoused by different sectors. In Chapter 3, MLVA noted her surprise when reading DH guidelines that referred to the health visitor's role as 'THE lead professional around early years . . . to instruct other people . . . there was no mention of partnership or collaboration.'

Greater awareness of the importance of *learning* rather than teaching has led to greater recognition that learners do not simply receive information. Individuals construct their own knowledge and understanding, combining new information with current and past experience. Constructivist approaches to learning form the basis of adult learning theory (Knowles 1984), an approach that currently informs professional education and underpins many methods of curriculum delivery such as problem- or enquiry-based learning. Medical education has now adopted more problem-based learning approaches, reducing its emphasis on codified bodies of knowledge (Stjernquist and Crang-Svalenius 2007). Such a change in approach to learning may encourage greater awareness of the influence of learners' prior experience on their construction of knowledge and understanding. Constructivist learning theory also encompasses narrative learning, an approach that sees learners as connecting to experience through reflection. Narrative learning theory argues that learners give meaning to experience through storytelling, which is seen as a natural human process of sense-making (Clark and Rossiter 2008). It is the emotional salience of stories about failure to protect the vulnerable that can be the most powerful prompts for individual and collective learning. Webb and Stimson (1976) used the term 'atrocity stories' in their research on doctor–patient consultations. They found that vivid accounts of experience served as 'a form of communication by which people make sense of past events', told in terms which allow the narrator to affirm their own integrity, and the integrity of the vulnerable. Li and Arber (2006) similarly use the term to explore nurses' accounts of troubled, credible patients in palliative care settings. Social worker(4) in Chapter 5 uses one such story to make sense of her learning from her own distress:

I was really . . . upset that the system had failed her and that I'd been naïve enough to presume that it was going on, so it was a learning curve for me . . . and there was an investigation and some of that came down to workload, but it left me really, really upset . . . some of that came down to letting each other know . . . if only they'd phoned me and left a message and e-mailed me to say we've changed our mind . . . and you've got to work through then how you feel towards your other professionals, which I found very hard for weeks . . . so there's a lot of learning curves . . . and it really is talking to one another, isn't it?

Despite the emphasis on adult learning, learning theories focusing on the individual have often relied on models of child development which can be relevant in the context of professional and interprofessional education. For example, literature on interprofessional learning has drawn on Piaget's (1958) work to introduce the concept of 'decentring'. In Piaget's stages of cognitive development, whereas the pre-operational child has a subjective and self-centred grasp of the world, the concrete operational stage is marked by the gradual waning of egocentricity and the development of the ability to 'decentre' or to consider multiple aspects of a situation simultaneously. This cognitive process supports awareness of points of view other than one's own, and an ability to 'think about thinking', one's own and others' (Clark 2006, Dahlgren 2006).

The voices in Part I recognize a clear link between learning practices and working practices. Eraut (2005) noted that neither educators nor practitioners give this link the attention it deserves. It is possible that such lack of attention has, in the past, stemmed from limitations in ways of understanding the relationship between theory and practice, formal and informal learning. Newer approaches to understanding experiential learning may help understand learning in complex interprofessional settings. These newer approaches adopt a social model of learning.

ACTIVITY

Reflect on your own preferred learning approaches and note down learning experiences you have particularly enjoyed or disliked. Can you identify any ways in which different approaches influence your current working practices?

Social learning theories

Communities of practice

The recognition that learning is a situated activity taking place in a social context is most clearly articulated by Lave and Wenger (1991). They identified that situated cognition facilitates learning from and through practice. Wenger (1998) theorized that new knowledge is created in communities of practice through active participation, defined as mutual engagement, joint enterprise and shared repertoire of discourses and techniques. Wenger sees the model of communities of practice as a social model of learning and of identity, distinguishing it from constructivist theory such as Piaget's that focuses on the learner's mental structures. In Wenger's model we define who we are by the ways we experience ourselves through participation in the various communities to which we belong, as well as the way we and others reify ourselves. Learners may often experience peripheral participation in a community of practice; their experiences may be affected by assumptions about the legitimacy of their participation. Wenger (1998) perceived novices as learning alongside experienced colleagues, moving from peripheral to full participation in a community. As Wenger (1998:152) suggests:

> when we are with a community of practice of which we are a full member, we are in familiar territory . . . we experience competence and we are recognised as competent, we know how to engage with others, we understand why they do what they do . . . moreover we share the resources they use to communicate.

Commentators on the notion of 'community of practice', however, have criticized its emphasis on collegiality and commonality at the expense of diversity (Eraut 2002) and its inability to embrace multiprofessional learning (Taylor 2004, Frost *et al.* 2005). Goodwin *et al.* (2005) used the notion of a community of practice to analyse interprofessional working in anaesthetics. They observed that learning experiences were controlled by senior staff (the consultant anaesthetist) according to perceptions of legitimate participation. Nurses' and operating department practitioners' participation in activities and hence their learning was more restricted than that of the trainee anaesthetists. Although interprofessional work groups may be able to create their own communities of practice, there is a danger that the potential for conformity inherent in the characteristics of a community of practice can be disempowering to newcomers.

Activity theory and expansive learning

Another social learning approach is activity theory, first developed by Vygotsky (1978), who introduced the idea of cultural mediation of actions. This suggested that 'the individual could no longer be understood without his or her cultural means; and the society could no longer be understood without the agency of individuals who use and produce artefacts' (Engeström 2001:134). Leont'ev (1981) developed Vygotsky's insights into a three-level model of activity. Object-related motive drives the uppermost level of collective activity; the middle level (of individual or group) is driven by a conscious goal and the bottom-level activity is framed by the conditions and tools (including ways of conceptualizing issues and tasks, as well as material objects) of the action. Engeström's further development of activity theory provides a conceptual and visual model to explore and understand the interrelationship between aspects of activity systems, but also particularly explores issues around knowledge creation and exchange. Engeström emphasized the multi-voiced nature of any activity system and the role of contradictions as sources of change, leading to the possibility of expansive learning and transformation. Contradictions inherent in any activity system will lead some individuals

> to question and deviate from its established norms. In some cases this escalates into collaborative envisioning and a deliberate collective change effort. An expansive transformation is accomplished when the object and motive of the activity are reconceptualised to embrace a radically wider horizon of possibilities than in the previous mode of the activity.
>
> (Engeström 2001:137)

The relevance of expansive learning for interprofessional working is obvious, and there is some evidence in Part I that organizational changes do reveal contradictions that lead to changing practices. The occupational therapist (OT1) in Chapter 1 seems to demonstrate an implicit understanding of the importance of the interrelationship between the social and organizational context of work and the activity of an integrated team. Office location is seen as significant in supporting team integration and opportunities for communication appear to provide valuable opportunities for informal learning, 'people are actually now thinking . . . how can you involve other people and help them feel more comfortable?' This change in thinking may have been facilitated by a change in organization and use of office space:

> When we first moved in people had psychology rooms and the OT room and it was disastrous, and it was a conscious thing on the teams when people left and we re-jigged the whole thing, the social workers came in recently so everybody moved offices . . . there's a social worker in each office . . . we have mixed professions in each office . . . everybody leaves the door open and so we have quite a lot of conversation, which is really helpful.

The importance of the organization of space is confirmed by Chapter 1's community nurse working in an intermediate care team who noted the effect of office reorganization on perceptions of support and on effective teamwork:

> We've just moved offices and prior to the move . . . the professionals were separated from the support workers and it was quite difficult . . . the last two months since we moved here have been wildly different . . . now, I would put [our interprofessional working] at 8/9 out of 10. It really is spot-on. The support workers feel much more supported and that they are being listened to.

Learning issues arising from workforce change

Models of support

All professions have a form of mentorship or supervision to support the neophyte professional. Part I illuminates a range of different models adopted by the different professions, but also considerable awareness of the importance of qualified staff as role models for students and junior colleagues. The ECC in Chapter 2 had explicit ideas about role modelling for interprofessional working, based on a non-hierarchical approach to professional collaboration.

> Emergency care is a low level in terms of prestige as a medical speciality. There's not too much of an ingrained hierarchy . . . the role modelling for the trainee is all about kind of integration, teamworking, etcetera, etcetera, and we work very hard with the trainees to look at communication skills, interpersonal working.

Obstetric consultant(2) in Chapter 4 also made it clear that she explicitly teaches junior doctors to respect midwives and their skills, noting, 'we say to our junior, the midwives know far more than you guys know, and you must respect them and defer to them, they're professionals in their own right'. Hafford-Letchfield *et al.* (2008:74) identify a range of facilitator skills important for supporting interprofessional learning in the workplace: 'the ability to be inclusive, facilitate across professional/worker groups, establish clear working agreements, handle conflict fairly, challenge constructively, avoid getting "professionally" defensive, take risks and deal with uncertainty'.

ACTIVITY

Can you identify your own role models for interprofessional working? What do you learn from them?

Reflect on yourself as a role model for interprofessional working. What do you think others learn from you?

One of the difficulties within interprofessional working is the lack of shared understanding of established support roles for learning. Whereas nursing students have qualified staff acting as mentors in practice settings, newly qualified staff should be supported by a period of preceptorship. Neither of these terms is familiar within social care. In social care supervision is seen as pivotal to achieving a quality service, with supervision seen as a bridge between line management and practitioners. In mental health settings, supervision is also a regular feature of professional practice. This worked particularly well in the unit for people with eating disorders (Chapter 5), and mental health nurse(1) saw the monthly supervision meetings as supportive of the team's collaborative activity. Such time is prioritized, and the ability to 'sit down with one another and discuss things' is seen as central to their success. In midwifery, however, all practitioners are required to have supervisors, but the supervisor's role does not have a strong educative and supportive function. Hence supervision is a term with varied meanings across professions.

Skills development

The challenge of effective collaborative working to ensure safe and effective service delivery brings its own challenges for initial and continuing professional education. Although there is widespread recognition of the importance of improving interpersonal and communications skills, there are justifiable concerns about the impact of current workforce change on professional education. A main direction of workforce change is to give senior professionals a stronger role in managing teams of support staff and a reduced role in direct care provision. Hence a doctor, in different settings, becomes responsible for the service provision, necessitating delegation of activities to other professional and support staff. Both the ECC and obstetric consultant(2) noted a concern about the impact on medical training of 'skilling up' other professionals, despite their explicit support for other professions taking on what had hitherto been seen as medical work. Junior doctors need time to gain skills and experience, and changing systems creates anxieties 'that medical staff don't get expertise . . . we are not entirely clear how we are training people for the future' (ECC). Hence concern about how one's own profession is developing skills can lead to restricting learning opportunities in the workplace, as illustrated in Goodwin *et al.*'s (2005) study of the anaesthetic team. In health care, the voices in Part I suggest that the attitude of senior medical staff plays a key role in facilitating or inhibiting workforce change.

The task of 'training up', that is, increasing the skill repertoire of staff, is generally supported by development of protocols that establish clear boundaries for decision making. Nevertheless, protocol-based care is also criticized for failing to develop autonomous decision-making and professional judgement. Goodwin *et al.* (2005) suggest that development of professional roles through protocol-based services will not improve service delivery because only medical trainees will be supported to gain and retain prescriptive and diagnostic capacities. The voices in Part I would not necessarily support this pessimistic view.

It is interesting that service user(1) in Chapter 3 is alert to the training needs of her personal assistants. She sends them on courses to develop particular skills such as manual handling and sees accepting some responsibility for training as part of her obligations as an employer, a role she voluntarily undertakes under the direct payment system. Service developments have identified a range of learning needs for the health and social care workforce. The community development worker, for example, notes that policy changes have ensured that 'people have had to learn more and more how to deal constructively with

---

ACTIVITY

Do you support students as part of your role? If so, reflect on your own strategies about supporting their learning. What opportunities do you provide for them to learn about or be assessed by professionals from other disciplines and by service users?

the voluntary sector'. This involves learning about inclusive and collaborative partnership working with communities, adopting approaches that are particularly unfamiliar to health professionals.

Does interprofessional learning make a difference to interprofessional working?

Over the past decade in the UK, there has been considerable interest in interprofessional education as one way of ensuring that professionals develop the skills for interprofessional collaboration. Interprofessional education, both pre- and post-qualification, has been widely introduced to improve professionals' knowledge about different professional roles, to enhance teamwork and communication skills and to promote positive attitudes towards working together and particularly towards working in partnership with the service user. Interprofessional education has grown, despite absence of clear evidence about the effectiveness of interprofessional learning in enhancing user-centred collaborative practice, and despite a lack of consensus on the question of when interprofessional learning (IPL) is most appropriate – pre- or post-registration. Despite the considerable logistical challenges in organizing interprofessional learning opportunities for large numbers of students, endorsement of the importance of IPL by the Quality Assurance Agency and by professional bodies has led to widespread implementation of IPL within pre-qualifying curricula (see for example Barrett *et al.* 2003, Hind *et al.* 2003, Lindquist *et al.* 2005, O'Halloran *et al.* 2006, Jackson and Bluteau 2007). The logistical challenges of bringing students together can partly be met through on-line learning, both through using shared e-resources and through collaborating on line. In the UK the Centre for Interprofessional e-learning (CIPeL) was established in 2005 with a remit to produce creative and innovative solutions to barriers to effective IPL. CIPeL has established a repository of learning objects (available from www.cipel.ac.uk/learning_objects/learning_objects.htm). The Social Care Institute for Excellence (SCIE) is also developing interactive electronic resources to support collaborative learning and teamworking (Thomas *et al.* 2009).

There is growing evidence about the effectiveness of interprofessional education. Hammick *et al.* (2007), reporting on evaluations of 15 pre-qualifying interprofessional initiatives that meet quality criteria for inclusion in a Best Evidence Medical Education systematic review, found that only two studies (Dienst and Byl 1981, Reeves and Freeth 2002) were able to demonstrate any impact of interprofessional learning on patient care. Nevertheless, a range of studies demonstrated some impact of pre-qualifying IPL on participants' knowledge, skills and attitudes, and Hammick *et al.* (2007) report evidence of effectiveness of postqualifying interprofessional learning initiatives from seven studies. Interprofessional learning initiatives have been shown to lead to improvements in screening or illness prevention services and Morey *et al.* (2002) found a reduction in observed medical errors among US teamwork trained emergency department staff. The editors of this book have conducted a longitudinal evaluation of pre-qualification interprofessional education among health and social care professions, following participants from entry to qualified practice. Qualified practitioners with IPL experience were more positive about their interprofessional relationships than practitioners on unipro-fessional curricula (Pollard and Miers 2008). Experience of IPL appeared to produce and sustain positive attitudes towards collaborative working. Newly registered medical doctors in Sweden exposed to IPL reported significantly more confidence that their studies had given them co-operative skills than newly qualified doctors without IPL experience (Faresjo *et al.* 2007). These results are encouraging and suggest that ending the tradition of 'silo' professional education may have a positive effect on the quality of interprofessional working.

ACTIVITY

Reflect on your experience of opportunities for learning with other professionals. How successful was it? What did you learn? Did the experience change your practice?

If so, in what ways? What might the facilitators have added to enhance the experience?

Summary

This chapter began by looking at the negative effects of separate cultures developing through professional socialization, an inevitable aspect of education. A brief overview of research into professional socialization is followed by a similarly brief overview of theories of learning. Successful interprofessional collaboration involves both understanding how the behaviour of professionals is influenced by their education and an ability to reflect on our own attitudes and actions and to learn from experience. Readers are encouraged to reflect on themselves as learners through the Activities. The chapter ends by considering the learning needs of a changing workforce and the potential of inter-professional education to develop collaborative skills.

References

Barbour RS (1985) Dealing with the transsituational demands of professional socialisation. *Sociological Review* 3:495–531.

Barrett G, Greenwood R, Ross K (2003) Integrating interprofessional education into 10 health and social care programmes. *Journal of Interprofessional Care* 17:293–301.

Barrett G, Sellman D, Thomas J (2005) *Interprofessional Working in Health and Social Care: Professional Perspectives – An Introductory Text.* Basingstoke:Palgrave Macmillan.

Barretti M (2004) What do we know about the professional socialisation of our students? *Journal of Social Work Education* 40(2):255–83.

CAIPE (1997) *Interprofessional Education: A Definition*. London:Centre for the Advancement of Interprofessional Education.

Carpenter J (1995) Doctors and nurses: stereotypes and stereotype change in interprofessional education. *Journal of Interprofessional Care* 9:151–61.

Carpenter J, Hewstone M (1996) Shared learning for doctors and social workers: evaluation of a programme. *British Journal of Social Work* 26:239–57.

Clark MC, Rossiter M (2008) Narrative learning in adulthood. *New Directions for Adult and Continuing Education* 119:61–70.

Clark P (2006) What would a theory of interprofessional education look like? Some suggestions for developing a theoretical framework for teamwork training. *Journal of Interprofessional Care* 20(6):577–89.

Coulehan J, Williams P (2001) Vanquishing virtue: the impact of medical education. *Academic Medicine* 76:598–604.

Dahlgren LO (2006) *Developing flexibility through experiencing variety: a potential function of interprofessional learning for improving competence*. Paper presented at the All Together Better Health III Conference: Challenges in Education and Practice, April, London.

DH (2000) *The NHS Plan: A Plan for Investment, a Plan for Reform*. Cmnd 4818-1, London:The Stationery Office.

Dienst ER, Byl N (1981) Evaluation of an educational program in health care teams. *Journal of Community Health* 6:282–98.

Dingwall R, Rafferty AM, Webster C (1988) *An Introduction to the Social History of Nursing*. London:Routledge.

Engeström Y (2001) Expansive learning at work: toward an activity theoretical reconceptualisation. *Journal of Education and Work* 14(1):133–56.

Eraut M (1994) *Developing Professional Knowledge and Confidence*. London and New York:Routledge Falmer.

Eraut M (2002) *Conceptual analysis and research questions: do the concepts of 'Learning Community' and 'Community of Practice' provide added value?* Paper presented at the Annual Conference of the American Educational Research Association, April, New Orleans.

Eraut M (2005) Editorial: Uncertainty in research. *Learning in Health and Social Care* 5(1):1–8.

Faresjo T, Wilhelmsson M, Pelling S, Dahlgren L-O, Hammer M (2007) Does interprofessional education jeopardize medical skills? *Journal of Interprofessional Care* 21(5):573–76.

Fox RC (1975) Training for uncertainty. In Cox C, Mead A (eds) *A Sociology of Medical Practice* London:Collier-Macmillan, 87–115.

Frost N, Robinson M, Anning A (2005) Social workers in multidisciplinary teams: issues and dilemmas for professional practice. *Child and Family Social Work* 10:187–96.

Goodwin C (1994) Professional vision. *American Anthropologist* 96(3):606–33.

Goodwin D, Pope C, Mort M, Smith A (2005) Access, boundaries and their effects: legitimate participation in anaesthesia. *Sociology of Health and Illness* 27(6):855–71.

Haas J, Saffir W (1977) The professionalization of medical students: developing competence and a cloak of competence. *Symbolic Interaction* 1(1):71–88.

Hafford-Letchfield T, Leonard K, Begum N, Chick NF (2008) *Leadership and Management in Social Care*. London:Sage.

Hall P (2005) Interprofessional teamwork: professional cultures as barriers. *Journal of Interprofessional Care* Supplement 1:188–96.

Hammick M, Freeth D, Koppel I, Reeves S, Barr H (2007) A best evidence systematic review of interprofessional education: BEME Guide no. 9. *Medical Teacher* 29(8):735–51.

Hawes D, Rees D (2005) Physiotherapy. In Barrett G, Sellman D, Thomas J (2005) *Interprofessional Working in Health and Social Care: Professional Perspectives – An Introductory Text*. Basingstoke:Palgrave Macmillan,109–18.

Hind M, Norman I, Cooper S, Gill E, Hilton R, Judd P, Jones SC (2003) Interprofessional perceptions of health care students. *Journal of Interprofessional Care* 17(1):21–34.

Jackson A, Bluteau P (2007) At first it's like shifting sands: setting up interprofessional learning within a secondary care setting. *Journal of Interprofessional Care* 21(3):351–3.

Knowles MS (1984) *Andragogy in Action: Applying Modern Principles of Adult Learning*. San Francisco:Jossey-Bass.

Lave J, Wenger E (1991) *Situated Learning: Legitimate Peripheral Participation*. Cambridge:Cambridge University Press.

Leont'ev AN (1981) *Problems of the Development of the Mind*. Moscow, Progress.

Li S, Arber A (2006) The construction of troubled and credible patients: a study of emotion talk in palliative care settings. *Qualitative Health Research* 16(1):27–46.

Lindquist SA, Duncan L, Shepstone L, Watts F, Pearce S (2005) Case-based learning in cross-professional groups: the development of a pre-registration interprofessional learning programme. *Journal of Interprofessional Care* 19(5):509–20.

Loseke DR, Cahill SE (1986) Actors in search of a character: student social workers' quest for professional identity. *Symbolic Interaction* 9:245–58.

Melia K (1987) *Learning and Working: The Occupational Socialisation of Nurses*. London:Tavistock.

Miers M (2000) *Gender Issues and Nursing Practice*. Basingstoke:Palgrave Macmillan.

Morey JC, Simon R, Jay GD, Wears RL, Salisbury M, Dukes KA, Berns SD (2002) Error reduction and performance improvement in the emergency department through formal teamwork training: evaluation results of the MedTeams project. *Health Services Research* 37:553–81.

NMC (2008) Confirmed principles to support a new framework for pre-registration nursing education. www.nmc-uk.org/aArticle.aspx?ArticleID=3396 (Accessed 04.03.2009).

O'Halloran C, Hean S, Humphris D, Macleod-Clark J (2006) Developing common learning: the new generation project undergraduate curriculum model. *Journal of Interprofessional Care* 19(3):251–68.

Petrie HG (1976) Do you see what I see? *Journal of Aesthetic Education* 10:29–43.

Piaget J (1958) *The Growth of Logical Thinking from Childhood to Adolescence*. New York:Basic Books.

Pollard KC (2008) Non-formal learning and interprofessional collaboration in health and social care: the influence of the quality of staff interaction on student learning about collaborative behaviour in practice placements. *Learning in Health and Social Care* 7(1):12–26.

Pollard KC, Miers ME (2008) From students to professionals: results of a longitudinal study of attitudes to pre-qualifying collaborative learning and working in health and social care in the United Kingdom. *Journal of Interprofessional Care* 22(4):399–416.

Reeves S, Freeth D (2002) The London training ward: an innovative interprofessional initiative. *Journal of Interprofessional Care* 16(1):41–52.

Stjernquist M, Crang-Svalenius E (2007) Problem based learning and the case method: medical students change preferences during clerkship. *Medical Teacher* 29 (8):814–20.

Taylor I (2004) Multiprofessional teams and the learning organisation. In Gould N, Baldwin M (eds) *Social Work, Critical Reflection and the Learning Organisation*. Aldershot:Ashgate, 75–86.

Thomas J, Whittington C, Quinney A (2009 forthcoming) *Working Collaboratively in Different Types of Teams* (available at www.scie.org.uk/publications/elearning/ipiac/index.asp (forthcoming).

Vygotsky LS (1978) *Mind in Society: The Development of Higher Psychological Processes*. Cambridge, MA:Harvard University Press.

Webb B, Stimson G (1976) People's accounts of medical encounters. In: Wadsworth M, Robinson E (eds) *Studies in Everyday Medical Life*. London:Martin Robertson,108–22.

Wenger E (1998) *Communities of Practice: Learning, Meaning and Identity*. Cambridge:Cambridge University Press.

Wilcock AA (2002) *Occupation for Health: A Journey from Self-health to Prescription*, Vol 2. London:British Association and College of Occupational Therapists.

Witz A (1992) *Professions and Patriarchy*. London:Routledge.

Individual and Professional Identity

Billie Oliver and Celia Keeping

Introduction: context and background

In 1999, the White Paper *Modernising Government* (Cabinet Office 1999) asserted that professional policy-making needed to change in order to respond to the 'increasingly complex, uncertain and unpredictable' world, and that to achieve this change it should be 'forward looking, outward looking, innovative and creative, questioning established ways and encouraging new ideas . . . inclusive . . . joined up . . . evaluative'. The advent of what is often described as 'joined-up' services means that interprofessional activity is required to meet multiple objectives and professionals are expected to work together and share their expertise and skills.

As illustrated by the experiences of the practitioners in Part I, this 'joined-up' approach can have positive outcomes and lead to greater effectiveness. For example in Chapter 2, the emergency care consultant (ECC) describes roles between nurses and doctors as being quite interchangeable around the issue of taking blood. At the same time, however, some may feel that the 'unique' skills they possess are effectively downgraded or lost (Tucker 2005). As Miller (2004:152) has argued, these calls for collaboration have come at the same time as many professionals 'feel threatened by a loss of identity and autonomy and are struggling to maintain a professional role'. Interprofessionalism, he suggests, has often been perceived as an attempt to 'de-professionalise or undermine professional legitimacy'. As we have seen in Part I, the overlap of roles and the perceived encroachment of traditional territory can lead to practitioners questioning their place within the interprofessional system. In

Chapter 1 the GP talks about practice nurses taking on more of a clinical role within GP surgeries and delegating less specialist tasks to health care assistants. This impacted on the role and identity of the doctors: 'Some doctors are a bit worried about this; I have heard doctors comment, "Where is this going to end; are these nurses trying to be doctors?"'

This permeability and interchangeability of roles can challenge the 'normative space' (Henkel, 2000:261) of practitioner values and can be experienced as a threat to their particular professional identity. The blurring of boundaries between professional roles as well as the often unspoken, yet powerful requirement to operate within new sets of values, rules and procedures as defined by the new partnership or interprofessional team may threaten the identity of distinct professional groups, each of whom relate to their own set of guiding ideals, ethical principles and rules (Banks 2004). Practitioners in single-profession, or single-agency, settings tend not to be required to justify the conceptual base of their actions or interactions. In a multi-agency or interprofessional setting, however, 'differences potentially collide as boundaries around specialisms are broken down' (Frost *et al.* 2005:189).

Frost *et al.* (2005:188) have observed how this blurring of professional knowledge boundaries can generate 'discomfort, anxiety and anger' as team members 'struggle to cope with the disintegration of one version of professional identity before a new version can be built'. Eraut (2004) has described this as a 'transition period' wherein practitioners cannot rely on their intuitive practice or tacit knowledge and will find their performance level reduced: 'The result is disorientation, exhaustion and vulnerability. The practitioners have become novices again without having the excuse of being a novice to justify a level of performance that fails to meet even their own expectations (p114).

Hunter (2003:333) has suggested that much existing research concerning the roles and identity of professionals has tended to be carried out within the context of 'changing notions of professional power, efficiency, competence and accountability', that is, in terms of what it is that makes 'a professional'. Freidson (1994:150), however, argues that 'whatever else a profession is, it represents a kind of work that people do for a living'. It is this construction of 'occupational identity' that is the focus of this chapter rather than the factors contributing to one's status as 'a professional'. What, for example, does calling oneself a 'social worker' or a 'nurse' mean in identity terms? And what happens to that sense of identity when the boundary between 'nurse' and 'social worker' becomes blurred through new integrated practices?

Lawler (2002:255) suggests that identity is not something which can be 'read off from an externally imposed schema'. People may well belong to designated groups – such as 'health visitor' or 'teacher' – but this in itself does not tell us about the kinds of individual identities that they build. Ibarra (1999:765) has argued, despite an apparent consensus in the literature, 'that identity changes accompany work role changes; the processes by which (professional) identity evolves remains under-explained'. It is hoped that this chapter will contribute to some understandings surrounding that process.

Postmodern analyses

Hall (1992:274) has suggested that a 'crisis of identity' is currently operating within 'modern societies' owing to the 'constant, rapid and permanent change' that is dislocating the central structures and processes of the social world. In essence, his argument is that the old identities which stabilized the social world for so long are in decline, giving rise to new and fragmented ones. Epstein (1978:101) argued that professional identity represents 'the process' by which a person seeks to 'integrate their various statuses and roles, as well as their diverse experiences, into a coherent image of self'. In the postmodern conceptualization it is this very process of identification that has 'become more open-ended, variable and problematic' (Hall 1992:276).

Hall (1992:275) discusses three different concepts of 'identity' debated within social theory. The 'Enlightenment Subject' was the traditional model for considering issues of identity and was based on an essentialist view of the individual having an 'inner core' that gradually unfolded throughout their life but which remained essentially the same. The emergence of the notion of the 'Sociological Subject' reflected the growing complexity of the modern world and the awareness that the 'inner core' was not 'autonomous and self sufficient, but was formed in relation to significant others'. The subject still has an 'inner core' or essence that is 'the real me' but this is formed and modified in a continuous dialogue with the cultural worlds 'outside'. Identity, in this conception, bridges the gap between the personal and the public worlds and 'stitches the subject into the structure'.

According to Hall, the subject is becoming fragmented, composed not of a single but of several sometimes contradictory or unresolved identities. In relation to professional identities Nixon (2003:12) follows Hall (1992) in suggesting that the changing context of practice has led to 'a runaway world' within which identity 'is never given; nor can it ever be achieved once and for all. It is always in the making'. Stronach *et al.* (2002) arrived at similar conclusions, rejecting the construct of 'a' professional identity such as 'a teacher' or 'a nurse' as being 'indefensibly unitary'. They reported finding that professionals frequently acknowledged a 'plurality of roles, uneasy allocations of priority, and uncertain attributions of identity' (p118). Furthermore, their plural accounts were far from stable. Professionals, they suggested, do not conduct their practices in the 'real' so much as they 'traffic between the twin abstractions of the ideal and the unrealised' (p132).

The agency/structural dichotomy

Halford and Leonard (1999) have asserted that two approaches to conceptualizing the relationship between work and identity have tended to dominate the literature. One of these sees individuals' distinctive identities developing as a consequence of their occupation; that is, that 'who we are' is constructed out of 'what we do' and that identity is etched onto individuals as they fill certain occupational roles. While personal choice may play some initial role in the choice of occupation, from that point onwards individuals develop distinctive identities as a consequence of their structural location within an organization or agency. The other perspective takes the view that individuals' innate and preformed identities are seen to determine the way in which work is carried out, so that 'what we do' is constructed out of 'who we are'. This approach views each of us as a unique soul. Here work is seen as an agentic activity – a way of expressing our 'true' identity. In this analysis the work we choose to do is a way of expressing our true self and we may seek out particular workplaces and/or occupations that enable us to 'be ourselves'. This structural/agentic dichotomy represents two ends of an argument but in reality both are needed to make sense of professional identity since both psychological and structural influences shape the individual from a very early stage in life.

Hoggett *et al.* (2006:699) argue that there does indeed exist an 'invariant core' or 'changing same' (Erikson 1968) within each of us which, while being subject to the influence of time and place, nevertheless changes only very slowly. This central core, they argue, is built up through a process of identifications with significant others in the child's early life. It is our analysis that these individual identities and the personal values that they give rise to play an important role in steering us towards our chosen professions and in contributing to the formation of our professional identities.

So the question of identity is a complex issue with multiple influences, both inner and outer, shaping how we see ourselves. With this in mind, therefore, the aim of this chapter is to explore some of the theoretical perspectives that attempt to explain the impact on professional identity of interprofessional working. In doing so we will examine a range of approaches to considering how individual and professional identities are formed, maintained and negotiated.

ACTIVITY

Can you identify a common strand or strands to the way in which you have constructed your identities that might be construed as a 'changing same'? What is the nature of that 'core' or 'changing same'? What have been some of the influences on you that have contributed to that'?

Identity and individual agency

Early influences

The study of early life and the place of identification in psychological development was pioneered by Freud and taken up later by Melanie Klein. In his later work, Freud (1921) claimed that identification with a significant other is the original form of emotional tie with an object and hence the basic building block of personal identity.

Following on from Freud, Klein believed that our relations with objects (that is, internal representation of figures and relationships which are emotionally significant, whether positively or negatively) comprise what we are on a most fundamental level and that the experience that the infant has of an internal object gives a sense of existence and identity. An internal object is created through a relationship between innate personal attributes and the external environment and depending on the quality of both it can be experienced as nurturing and loving or vengeful and persecuting. This object contributes to the foundations of the child's developing personality and since all of us are made up of both 'good' and 'bad' objects, one's identity can comprise both positive and negative attributes. Central to the concept of identity, however is the idea of relationship with others.

Winnicott (1971) developed this idea further when he referred to the mother's role in providing a 'mirror' for the infant in her responsiveness to the many moods and feelings, or 'imaginings' of the baby. By providing this quality of attention she is giving the baby an experience of recognition which is key to the baby's development of a sense of self. The basic building blocks of our identity can be thus very hard to change. Furthermore, because these identifications have their origins in the pre-thinking stage of our development, much is lost to conscious awareness and we may find it very difficult to fully understand who we are and why we may act in the way we do.

Adolescence

While the foundations of our identity are established during earlier stages of development, the period of adolescence tends to be characterized by a more conscious exploration of identity issues. Erikson (1968) viewed the adolescent's search for a personal identity as including the formation of a personal ideology or a philosophy of life that could provide a frame of reference for evaluating events. In this sense a personal identity is based on a personal philosophy that may influence the value orientation of the individual and consequently their choice of occupation (Muus 1996).

Erikson (1968), however, was the first to propose a 'life-span theory' of identity development within which he argued that the search for an identity was a continuing process but is constantly lost and regained through a process of questioning, exploration and commitment. It was Erikson's analysis that one's ability to cope with later life identity issues may well depend on the degree of success with which one mastered the adolescent identity crisis.

Moving into work

Hoggett (2005:5) drew similar conclusions, reporting that professionals often 'bring something to their work role in terms of values, identities and emotional capacities which pre-exists their engagement in that role'. He hypothesized that this was a significant factor in the ability of some practitioners to demonstrate resilience when negotiating what he calls the 'dilemmatic spaces' created by the introduction of new initiatives, such as interprofessional teams (p4). Values, Hoggett suggests, provide us a 'kind of compass' and help with our 'orientation' during exploration of new roles (p7).

In her study of the impact of interprofessional working within mental health services, Keeping (2006) also found a strong link between respondents' own personal values and the values which were described as being central to their profession, that of social work. Personal experiences were very often described as the motivating force behind respondents' entry into social work and fuelled their adherence to particular values. In many cases social workers were clear that specific incidents in their own lives had directly resulted in their choice of profession. Often this was found to be driven by a desire to redress significant and difficult earlier life experiences.

ACTIVITY

Reflect on some of the reasons why you chose your particular profession or role.

What are some of the personal values and/or life history events that drove that choice?

Identity and structural influences

Integrated children's services

In recent years, a considerable amount of the interprofessional change agenda has been aimed at integrating and reforming children's and young people's services. In 2003, the Laming inquiry set up to investigate the death of Victoria Climbié made a series of recommendations that led to the publication of *Every Child Matters* (DfES 2003). Laming (2003) concluded that children's needs were being neglected or overlooked through a lack of 'joined-up' working, poor systems for information sharing and too great a reliance on professional and agency boundaries. Hence, *Every Child Matters* was characterized by calls for the creation of new services and new working practices that emphasized the integration of services through multi-agency working and partnerships between the voluntary, community and statutory sectors including common assessments, information sharing and joint training. What has since become known as the '*Every Child Matters* agenda' has led to a comprehensive and radical review of approaches to the delivery of all children's and young people's services.

Laming (2009) has revisited many of the concerns raised in his earlier report (Laming 2003). One of the key strategic aims continues to stress that those working with children and young people should be enabled to work across professional boundaries (DfES 2005). The *Children's Workforce Strategy* (DfES 2005) set out a vision of a 'competent, confident and stable' workforce that would 'overcome the restrictive impact of professional and organizational boundaries'. It aimed to achieve this through 'stimulating new ways of working and the development of new roles' and through the introduction of a single qualifications framework built around the 'common core of skills and knowledge'.

Every Child Matters was followed, very swiftly, by the passing of the *Children Act* (Great Britain 2004), which introduced legislation to establish strategic partnerships, called Children's Trusts, in every local authority. This consequent restructuring of local authority services for children and young people is now well under way, for example in Chapter 3 the manager of a large voluntary agency (MLVA) discusses experience of participating in a Children's Trust. However, a study commissioned by the DfES to 'explore and evaluate the key issues emerging in moving towards Children's Trust processes' reported that the most common 'issue' was 'to do with the workforce'. 'Some . . . staff were said to be resisting change and were even in denial of what the transition actually meant' (ECOTEC 2006:6). A subsequent report found that progress in integrating children's services into Children's Trusts had been hampered by a 'lack of clarity about purposes and frameworks' and that 'there has been a lot of legislation and guidance, but a failure to communicate the changing emphasis effectively' (Audit Commission 2008:10–11). The MLVA illustrates this frustration when she describes how 'some Trust members had quite boundaried roles, others had more autonomy, others were not able to make any decisions and had to take things back for further consultation. This could make things quite cumbersome.'

Halford and Leonard (1999) suggest that the 'majority' of change management initiatives work from a 'structural' interpretation such as this, with organizations trying to 'bend individual identities to their own imperatives' while failing to take sufficient account of the individual or collective values that underpin many people's professional identities. They argue that this approach often leads to individuals 'resisting or circumventing' the imposed changes in order to maintain their own identities. This is illustrated in Chapter 1 when the health visitor expresses her struggles with current changes:

> There's been a lot of change and a lot of insecurity, so health visitors are . . . desperately trying to hold on to what they know they can do, and not wanting others to do assessments for them, etcetera, keeping that responsibility. And that's quite difficult when you've got a multiprofessional team, and you're meant to be working together.

Halford and Leonard (1999) concluded that change cannot take place in the abstract, independent of the individuals who constitute the organization. They found that rather than take on a new identity through 'labelling from above', individuals appear to take a 'more agentic role in evaluating (the ideologies) and placing themselves in relation to it'. Change, they argue, depends, in part, on the identification of staff with the new values and priorities. In other words, change will only take place if individuals 'live out' or 'embody' the new practices (p107).

In Chapter 3 the MLVA describes challenges she encountered around the clash of professional values in relation to children's involvement: 'Different professional groups have very different understanding, experiences and attitudes around participation and there can be tensions around this.'

Social identity theory

In identity theory, the core of an identity is said to be the 'categorisation of the self as an occupant of a role, and the incorporation, into the self, of the meanings and expectations associated with that role and its performance' (Stets and Burke 2000:225). These expectations and meanings are said to form a set of standards that guide our behaviour in role. In Social Identity Theory, an individual does not have one 'personal self', but rather several selves that correspond to the groups to which they belong. In this analysis each group has its own social identity and uniqueness as opposed to each person's unique identity. People have as many different social identities as there are groups to which they feel they belong.

Implicit within social identity theory are assumptions that individuals gain self-esteem from social groups and so will pursue goals that maintain or increase their social or collective identity. Studies have indicated that at times of organizational change and restructuring individuals often display strong inter-group behaviour that inhibits a new collective identity (Haunschild *et al.* 1994). Subjective comparisons between the old and the new organizational or professional identities are made, and if the new one appears superior, then individuals are more likely to abandon their old identities and accept the new one. However, if the new identity seems inferior in any way, then the employees may hold on to their old identities and reject the new.

In Chapter 1 the health visitor illustrates this emotional response when she refers to 'these lower-paid people coming in, and a health visitor post goes'. This results in 'a lot of insecurity' with health visitors 'desperately trying to hold on to what they know they can do'. Similarly, in Chapter 4 community midwife(2) describes feeling 'outnumbered by the health visitors' resulting in her feeling 'condescended to' and a 'kind of rivalry' emerging.

Othering

In Chapter 1 the GP suggests feeling 'elbowed out' by the 'more organized' midwives and feeling that a situation of 'us and them' exists with social workers in the team. When people categorize themselves as a member of a group, similarities in the group and differences between the 'in-group' and 'out-group' are accentuated. An important aspect of the process of social categorization is that of 'othering' – of perceiving groups of people as being different to other groups. The concept of 'othering' is an important one in the formation of both an individual and a group identity and is defined in terms of what is taken to be 'self' in contrast to what is considered to be 'other'. The means by which one differentiates oneself from others is considered to be central to the experience of forming an identity (Geldard and Geldard 2004). The process of 'othering' is seen as a way of defining and securing one's own positive identity through the stigmatization of an 'other'.

The relationship between subject and 'othered' object can imply an unequal distribution of power, whereby the object is defined by and in relation to the person or group occupying the subject position. For instance, according to de Beauvoir (1949), women have been turned into an objectified 'other' by men who have claimed the subject position themselves, thereby appropriating the power to define and dominate women. Professional groups who lack the power to assert their own position within an interprofessional team could be at risk of being placed in the position of 'other', thereby jeopardizing their independence and the power to define themselves.

In Part I we can observe some evidence of this process of constructing 'others' between professional groups. For example, in Chapter 2 the physiotherapist suggests that the nurses in their team have 'completely different values', and in Chapter 3 the MLVA expresses the belief that 'different professional groups have 'very different understandings, experiences and attitudes around participation'.

ACTIVITY

Reflect on some of the situations when you have been in an interprofessional team. Did you feel differently about your identity/role than you do when in a group with people from the same profession/background as yourself? What was the nature of that difference and how did it make you feel/act? For example: did it make you feel more or less comfortable; more or less knowledgeable? What contributory factors do you attribute to this?

Basic assumptions

As we have seen, individuals are drawn to particular professions for complex reasons, some of which may be beyond their conscious awareness. In so doing, their personal identity becomes reinforced by their social identity and a strong professional identity is formed. Bion (1961) found that different professional groups use particular defensive processes, what he called 'basic assumptions' which draw on particular emotions, values and ideas in relation to their main task. These defences are ways of dealing with difficult emotions in response to, for instance, organizational change and internal conflict between managers and employees or between different professional groups. Where groups utilizing different basic assumptions come together, as in interprofessional teams for example, there can be a clash of philosophies with a resultant threat to the identity of the less powerful professional group.

In Chapter 1 we saw that the prevailing philosophy of the integrated community team, as described by Occupational therapist(1), appears to be that of the medical model, based on the idea of individual pathology and dependency on the expertise of clinicians. Despite a name change to that of 'service users' meeting', the regular clinical meeting, with its emphasis on the 'patient/clinician' dyad, continues to be a source of discomfort to the social workers who may well subscribe to a different model of care. Finding themselves in this philosophically alien territory could pose a threat to social work identity and could result in further defensive activity, impeding the collaborative work of the team.

Community identity

Adams and Marshall (1996) have pointed out the apparent 'paradoxical association' between two 'seemingly opposing factors': the need for a sense of uniqueness or individuation and the need for 'communion' which focuses on the need for 'belongingness, connectedness, and union with others'. They have argued that identity construction is dependent on both a sense of uniqueness and a sense of belonging and that the dynamic interplay between them is critical. Integration centres on the involvement, connection and communion with others and socialization that facilitates integration will result in 'a sense of mattering in the form of a social or collective identity' (p431). Too high a degree of differentiation, which results in 'extreme uniqueness' of an individual, can be met with a lack of acceptance by, and communion with, others, which can lead to marginalization. Conversely, 'extreme connectedness' and low differentiation can curtail an individual's sense of uniqueness and agency which can lead to difficulties adapting to new circumstances. These ideas have considerable significance to our discussion of professional identities and the role of communities of practice within changing practice contexts.

There has recently been a developing interest in Wenger's notion of 'communities of practice' and their relationship to the sustainability of professional identities. Wenger's work has been explored in Chapter 6, but has particular significance for understanding identity. Wenger (1998) suggested that there is an interactive and dynamic interplay between the identities of individuals and the communities to which they are affiliated. An individual's identity is not only shaped by the community, but that individual's identity can also shape and change the nature of that community.

Challenged identities

Ibarra (1999) has described the process of adjustment in a new role as the quest for a 'provisional self'. In her analysis, she was drawing on a theory developed by Markus and Nurius (1986) called the 'possible selves construct'. This theory built on Erikson's (1968) conclusion that the individual is continuously engaged in a quest for a stable identity and suggested that identity formation is influenced by an individual's ideas 'about what they might become, what they would like to become, and what they are afraid of becoming' (p954). Gilligan (2000:38) also drew on the notion of 'possible selves', arguing that developing an identity involves developing a sense of 'worthiness' and competence and that this, in turn, involves some comparison by the individual between how they would like to be and how they think they actually measure up.

Ibarra (1999) used the 'possible selves' construct to explore the processes through which people adapt to and grow into new career roles. She found that individuals experimented with 'provisional selves' that served as trials for possible, but not yet fully elaborated, professional identities. She concluded that individuals explored and tested out potential or 'provisional' identities in an iterative, cyclical fashion, continuously 'figuring out how to transfer old preferences and values to new and different contexts and how to integrate those with changing priorities' (Ibarra 2003:163). In describing what she called 'true-to-self strategies' for testing out 'provisional selves', Ibarra drew attention to 'the role of individual agency' in constructing identities. She found that a dominant theme in the experiences of her research participants was the degree of congruence between 'their provisional constructions' and 'conceptions of the kind of professional they were and aspired to be'. Many of her interviewees reported having taken on a structural identity associated with the organization or institution within which they had been working. In many cases, the 'reinvention' process they underwent involved breaking free from this identity to rediscover their 'possible selves'.

ACTIVITY

Can you identify other 'possible selves' that you might have tried out as you developed your professional identity? What have been some of the processes that you have experienced as helpful/unhelpful in deciding whether to reject or develop your emergent identity?

Moving forward

The refinement of identity, therefore, is continuous in response to particular psychosocial conditions, but the basic building blocks of personality laid down in early infancy remain. The resulting adult identity is thus heavily influenced by both personal relationships as well as social context in terms of expectations of self and others, values and needs, and this in turn influences the kind of work sought by the individual. This raises the question of whether it is ever possible to escape the impact of early influences on our identity.

Hoggett *et al.* (2006) draw on the work of Steiner (1996) to argue that in order to continue growing and developing in life – and this could include the requirement to adapt to new roles at work – something in us must die, the 'something' in question being the influence of early identifications. However, change does not necessarily mean the complete abandonment of an original identity, and good aspects may continue to contribute to our lives. Taylor (2004:86) has suggested that the process of transition into a new professional role and identity involves undergoing a period of 'unlearning'. Taylor suggests that practitioners must 'unlearn' before they can be effectively open to new practices and that the most effective way to achieve this is within a 'safe environment with informed, trusted and engaged colleagues'. In order for the interprofessional enterprise to be successful, a climate of reflexive awareness of our own personal motivations and identifications is necessary so that we retain the positive aspects of our own different professional identities, while understanding and addressing any unhelpful and obstructive aspects in our relations with other professional groups.

An example of 'unlearning' can be seen in the description by obstetric consultant(2) in Chapter 4 of 'newish junior doctors' who insist on treating the midwives

> as nurses to do exactly as he tells them, as the doctor; but it's never the kind of permanent staff that are here, you know we do not tolerate that, and we say to our juniors, the midwives know far more than you guys know, and you must respect them and defer to them, they're professionals in their own right.

=== **ACTIVITY** ===

Have you yourself experienced 'unlearning' and/or 'refocusing' when in interprofessional situations? What do you think has been positive about this?

Connected identities

Oliver (2007) found that recent initiatives to introduce 'joined-up' and interprofessional working mean that we need to view the concept of professional identity as a 'moveable feast' (Hall 1992). Hall (1992:275) has suggested that 'identity' only becomes an issue when it is in crisis, 'when something assumed to be fixed, coherent and stable is displaced by the experience of doubt and uncertainty'. Oliver (2007) has argued that a state of 'crisis' has been precipitated by the introduction of new roles and new working practices that have no established guidelines, boundaries or communities of practice. The impact of this crisis on pre-existing identities can be to generate feelings of loss, uncertainty, betrayal, disrespect and marginalization. The analysis of the 'Connected

Identity' (Oliver, 2007) takes the view that professional identity is dynamic and constantly in the process of being reconstructed as discourses on practice change. Importantly, also, this analysis maintains that change is not about abandoning a previous identity; rather it is about transforming it.

Oliver (2007) argues that when confronted with a challenge to personal and professional values practitioners are, in fact, often revisiting their 'forgotten selves': exploring how their preferred style and values relate to the new and different contexts. This appears to support Erikson's (1968) view that during the process in which a sense of identity develops or transforms there will be an unconscious striving for continuity with a previous sense of self.

The process of revisiting one's 'forgotten self' can often involve the practitioner in seeking out what Oliver (2007) calls 'like-minded others' – other practitioners striving to explore the values and principles behind their role – and that this can lead to the development of dynamic communities that cross traditional boundaries. For example Occupational therapist(1) (Chapter 1) suggests that, over time, the team ended up moulding their manager as they regained strength from asserting their knowledge and experience values. Whereas 'initially people were quite defensive' now 'they are trying to be more positive, to try and mould things and change things around'.

Adams and Marshall (1996:432) have argued that there can be a dynamic interplay between an individual's identity and the community to which they affiliate. If the balance between 'differentiation' and 'sameness' is right these cross-boundary interactions can result in exchanges which facilitate the adaptive evolution of both the individual and the group identity.

Summary

In this chapter we have presented a broad overview of a range of theoretical approaches to considering issues of identity construction, maintenance and transition within an interprofessional framework. A strong theme to emerge from many of these approaches is that the very idea of 'identity' is in a state of flux, owing to the constant and ongoing change that is challenging the central structures of our social world. As Hall (1992) has suggested, there is a continuous sense of incompleteness about our identities. They are always 'in process of being formed' (p287). In the context of this turmoil, attention has begun to focus on the factors that can contribute to the maintenance of a more resilient sense of identity. As we can see in many of the comments of the practitioners in Part I, the development of cross-boundary 'communities of practice' can provide the opportunities for exploration of our (not recently revisited) values and can lead to a reinvigorated sense of identity and consequently, practice.

The key points of the chapter include:

■ interprofessional teamwork can lead to the blurring of professional knowledge boundaries and professional identity can become challenged as roles and responsibilities change,

- the concept of 'identity' cannot be conceived of as fixed or permanent but as constantly being formed and re-formed as the discourse surrounding practice develops,

- values and individual agency act as a 'beacon' to guide us and help us make sense of challenges to our identity during times of change,

- interprofessional communities can provide opportunities for exploration of our values and identities and can lead to a reinvigorated practice.

References

Adams GR, Marshall SK (1996) A developmental social psychology of identity: understanding the person-in-context. *Journal of Adolescence* 19:429–42.

Audit Commission (2008) *Are We There Yet? Improving Governance and Resource Management in Children's Trusts*. London:Audit Commission.

Banks S (2004) *Ethics, Accountability and the Social Professions*. Basingstoke:Palgrave Macmillan.

Bion W (1961) *Experiences in Groups*. London:Tavistock.

Cabinet Office (1999) *Modernising Government*. London:The Stationery Office.

de Beauvoir S (1949) *The Second Sex*. Tr. HM Parshley. Harmondsworth:Penguin.

DfES (2003) *Every Child Matters*. London:The Stationery Office.

DfES (2005) *Children's Workforce Strategy: A Strategy to Build a World-class Workforce for Children and Young People*. Nottingham:DfES Publications.

ECOTEC (2006) *Connexions Moving Towards Children's Trusts: A Report to the Department for Education and Skills*. London:ECOTEC.

Epstein A (1978) *Ethos and Identity*. London:Tavistock.

Eraut M (2004) Learning to change and/or changing to learn. *Learning in Health and Social Care* 3(3):111–17.

Erikson EH (1968) *Identity: Youth and Crisis*. New York:Norton.

Freidson E (1994) *Professionalism Reborn: Theory, Prophecy and Policy*. Chicago:Polity Press.

Freud S (1921) Group psychology and the analysis of the ego. Tr. J Strachey. In: Strachey J (ed) (1955) *The Standard Edition of the Complete Psychological Works of Sigmund Freud, Volume XVIII (1920–1922)*. London:The Hogarth Press and the Institute of Psychoanalysis, 67–144.

Frost N, Robinson M, Anning A (2005) Social workers in multidisciplinary teams: issues and dilemmas for professional practice. *Child and Family Social Work* 10:187–96

Geldard K, Geldard D (2004) *Counselling Adolescents*. (2nd edn) London:Sage.

Gilligan R (2000) Adversity, resilience and young people: the protective value of positive school and spare time experiences. *Children & Society* 14:37–47.

Great Britain (2004) *Children Act*. London:The Stationery Office.

Halford S, Leonard P (1999) New identities? Professionalism, managerialism and the construc-tion of self. In: Exworthy M, Halford S (eds) *Professionals and the New Managerialism in the Public Sector*. Buckingham:Open University Press,102–20.

Hall S (1992) The question of cultural identity. In: Hall S, Held D, McGrew T (eds) *Modernity and Its Futures*. Cambridge:Polity Press, 273–325.

Haunschild PR, Moreland RL, Murrell AJ (1994) Sources of resistance to mergers between groups. *Journal of Applied Social Psychology* 24:1150–78.

Henkel M (2000) *Academic Identities and Policy Change in Higher Education*. London:Jessica Kingsley.

Hoggett P (2005) *Negotiating Ethical Dilemmas in Contested Communities.* ESRC End of Award Report, ref. RES-000–23–0127. www.esrcsocietytoday.ac.uk.

Hoggett P, Beedell P, Jimenez L, Mayo M, Miller C. (2006) Identity, life history and commitment to welfare. *Journal of Social Policy* 35(4):689–704.

Hunter S (2003) A critical analysis of approaches to the concept of social identity in social policy. *Critical Social Policy* 23(3):322–45.

Ibarra H (1999) Provisional selves: experimenting with image and identity in professional adaptation. *Administrative Science Quarterly* 44(4):764–91.

Ibarra H (2003) *Working identity: unconventional strategies for reinventing your career.* Boston:Harvard Business School Press.

Keeping C (2006) *Emotional Aspects of the Professional Identity of Social Workers: A Study of Social Workers Working within Avon and Wiltshire Mental Health Partnership NHS Trust.* University of the West of England, Bristol and Avon and Wiltshire Mental Health Partnership NHS Trust:Bristol.

Klein M, Riviere J (1964) *Love, Hate and Reparation.* New York:WW Norton.

Laming, Lord (2003) *Inquiry into the Death of Victoria Climbié.* London:The Stationery Office.

Laming, Lord (2009) *The Protection of Children in England: A Progress Report.* London:The Stationery Office.

Lawler S (2002) Narrative in social research. In: May T (ed) *Qualitative Research In Action.* London:Sage, 242–58.

Markus H, Nurius P (1986) Possible selves. *American Psychologist* 41:954–69.

Miller C (2004) *Producing Welfare; A Modern Agenda.* Basingstoke:Palgrave Macmillan.

Muus R (1996) *Theories of Adolescence.* New York:McGraw Hill.

Nixon J (2003) Professional renewal as a condition of institutional change: rethinking academic work. *International Studies in Sociology of Education* 13(1):3–15.

Oliver B (2006) Identity and change: youth working in transition. *Youth & Policy* 93:5–19.

Oliver B (2007) *Connected identities: professional identity in transition.* EdD thesis, University of Sussex, Brighton.

Steiner J. (1996) The aim of psychoanalysis in theory and practice. *International Journal of Psychoanalysis* 77:1073–83.

Stets JE, Burke PJ (2000) Identity theory and social identity theory. *Social Psychology Quarterly* 63(3):224–37.

Stronach I, Corbin B, McNamara O, Stark S, Warne T (2002) Towards an uncertain politics of professionalism: teacher and nurse identities in flux. *Journal of Education Policy* 17(1):109–38.

Taylor I (2004) Multi-professional teams and the learning organisation. In: Gould N, Baldwin M (eds) *Social Work, Critical Reflection and the Learning Organisation.* Aldershot:Ashgate, 75–86.

Tucker S (2005) The sum of the parts: exploring youth working identities. In: Harrison R, Wise C. (eds) *Working With Young People.* London:Sage, 204–12.

Wenger E (1998) *Communities of Practice: Learning, Meaning and Identity.* Cambridge:Cambridge University Press.

Winnicott D (1971) *Playing and Reality.* London:Tavistock/Routledge.

Professional Boundaries and Interprofessional Working

Margaret Miers

Introduction

An emphasis on developing skills in interprofessional working among the health and social care workforce is part of a policy agenda to develop a flexible workforce responsive to the needs of a rapidly changing service. The introductory chapter to this book has already identified a range of factors driving service change, including the rising expectations of knowledgeable and discerning individuals with experience of health and social care. Finch (2000:1129–30) has argued that Department of Health policy documents suggest the NHS 'wants students to be prepared for interprofessional working' for a range of reasons, including ensuring new entrants are 'able to "substitute for" roles traditionally played by other professionals when circumstances suggest that this would be effective' and to ensure that new entrants have career flexibility, involving 'moving across' traditional role boundaries. Such flexibility, centred on role substitution and role redesign, can present a challenge to professionals accustomed to established patterns of professional roles and professional boundaries. The accepted understanding of a 'profession' in health care has encompassed an expectation of autonomy, self-regulation and status conferred by distinctive areas of expertise, albeit organized around a hierarchical, medically led division of labour (Freidson 1970). Role redesign involves changing the division of labour and can change accepted patterns of power and authority. Hence the move to a more flexible workforce has attracted considerable exploration and analysis, particularly within sociological theory concerning professions and professionalization. This chapter draws on this literature to explore the tensions that can derive from changing professional boundaries. It draws on the insights Part I offers into the challenges, success and advantages of role redesign.

Some of the voices in Part I see flexibility around role boundaries as an intrinsic part of successful interprofessional working. An Occupational therapist (OT)(1), working in an integrated team for people with learning difficulties, for example, reports considerable overlap with physiotherapists in some activities, such as provision of walking aids and specialist seating. Despite the 'blurred barriers', she/he reports: 'I don't think anybody in the team feels really threatened by it' (see Chapter 1). In this integrated team (see later discussion), allocation of work is resolved through team discussion, and OT(1) reports, 'we mix people's skills'. Similarly, in Chapter 5, mental health nurse(1), working in a unit for people with eating disorders, reports that ways of working that allow individual professionals to 'pick and mix skills' are beneficial to team functioning and to service users. He reports that ' . . . although we do recognise boundaries and certain strengths . . . at certain points . . . we come together around them rather than fall apart because of them'.

In these examples, the organization of work involves using and developing individual strengths. Although such strengths may have been nurtured through experience in a professional role, traditional professional jurisdictions do not constrain individual contributions and this flexibility across boundaries is seen as a feature of effective interprofessional working.

In many settings, professionals contributing to Part I see flexibility around role boundaries as essential. In Chapter 1, a community nurse working in an intermediate home care team reports that involving 'each other in whatever aspects of care we are providing' is a normal part of daily work. Hence nurses will 'follow up programmes that the therapists set' and 'physios carry basic gloves and maybe a basic tape and gauze' to 'patch' wounds if necessary. Such flexibility avoids 'two or three different people' attending a client on one day. It is the client who benefits. The emergency care consultant (ECC) (Chapter 2) identifies role flexibility, particularly around medical and nursing boundaries, as essential for creating a safe environment.

> If the medical staff are busy, the nursing staff take blood. If the nursing staff are busy, the medical staff take blood . . . what's important is that somebody does it and it fits into the overall workload of the department.

The senior registrar, paediatrics (SRP) like the ECC, is entirely comfortable with changing role boundaries and is 'all for everybody getting extra training and doing things differently, because it's more efficient for the patient'.

Nevertheless, some professionals voice concerns about role overlap and changes in professional boundaries. In Chapter 1 the GP notes that midwives' autonomy as the professional responsible for normal labour 'is a point of contention as the GP's role is much less than it used to be'. This change had led to GPs who were 'very hot on obstetrics' feeling they had lost expertise 'as if you don't use your skills, particularly in obstetrics, you get rusty'. Doctors felt 'elbowed out'. They are losing areas of work in which they gained satisfaction from exercising their own expertise. The health visitor in Chapter 1 also reports tensions around the introduction of new roles and changing boundaries. Skill mix, the health visitor explains, 'has always been seen as a threat, because you have these lower-paid people coming in, and a health visitor post goes'. In contrast to the SRP who perceived changing role boundaries as an opportunity for all to gain more training to work in different ways, the health visitor described negative aspects of change. Policy initiatives such as Sure Start have introduced a

> play worker, the community nurse, the health visitor assistants, etcetera. Whereas before there was just a health visitor, with maybe a health visitor assistant. It was brought in, and it wasn't made explicit, and it was seen as a watering-down rather than a boosting-up

Health visitors feel 'they're not being recognized'. Feelings of insecurity lead to a situation in which

> health visitors are . . . desperately trying to hold on to what they know they can do...and that's quite difficult when you've got a multiprofessional team, and you're meant to be working together.

Chapter 7 has attributed much of this anxiety to perceived threats to professional identity. Drawing on different understandings of 'identity' Oliver and Keeping explain how workforce change can disrupt individuals' sense of meaning and purpose. Chapter 10 reviews the significance of boundaries from varied perspectives on organizational theory. This chapter, in contrast, looks more closely at the boundary and workforce change in relation to the social position of professions and the social organization of professional work, exploring the challenge changes in perceived power relationships can pose for interprofessional working.

ACTIVITY

Role redesign and role expansion is common in health and social care services. Have such changes affected your own role and those of your colleagues in your workplace? Have any new roles been introduced?

Reflect on your own and colleagues' responses to such changes.

The 'problem' of professional power and professionalising projects

Sociological literature helps explain why tensions around overlapping and changing role boundaries may occur. In the UK, the analysis of professions has been heavily influenced by Freidson's work which identified the key characteristics of a profession as autonomy over work, specialized knowledge and expertise, control over entry and training and self-regulation. Freidson (1970) also identified medical dominance as the supreme exemplar of professional power. Health professions working alongside doctors have sought to develop their own areas of specialized expertise and to gain control over their own education and to maintain their own professional register in order to increase their status and power (Abbott 1988, Dingwall 1983, Witz 1992). Professional power has, however, been under considerable threat over recent decades through processes of managerialism and marketization introduced to control costs of providing services (Harrison 2002). Haug (1973) used the concept of deprofessionalization to depict a loss of professions' monopoly over knowledge and a loss of public belief in the credibility of professional expertise. McKinlay and Stoekle (1988) identified 'proletarianisation' as a threat to medical power, predicting salaried employment of doctors and deskilling of their professional practice through separating activities involved in patient care in order to allocate tasks to lower-paid employees. Devolving care to support workers can be seen as one such example. Professional power has also declined through the requirement to adhere to national guidance rather than use own individual judgement and experience in making decisions about patients. The GP in Chapter 1 comments that

> the days when you could make up what you think and play it as you want are no longer, and you really do have to follow the guidelines.

It is against this background of 'attack' that professionals respond to changes in ways of working. Lupton (1997) has argued that, in the case of medicine, both doctors and the public have no doubt that doctors are 'professionals' but changes in practice involve '*re*professionalisation'. Doctors in Lupton's study agreed that doctors were not 'as omnipotent as perhaps they once were' (p490). Reprofessionalization may involve accepting changing boundaries. Although GPs felt 'elbowed out' of maternity care, the GP identifies a range of activities that have been passed on to other professionals. In this GP's practice, passing on responsibility for cervical smear tests and devolving care of minor injuries to nursing staff did not lead to tension. Nevertheless she is aware of professional rivalry, noting, 'I have heard doctors comment, "Where is this going to end, are these nurses trying to be doctors?"'

Professional rivalry can be understood through the Weberian concept of social closure. Professions can be seen not as occupations with a privileged place in society because of the rarity and importance of their expertise for the general good, but as occupations seeking to gain advantageous positions in the labour market. Closure theory depicts a process whereby occupations as social collectivities act to ensure their status and rewards in society are protected, usually by restricting access to the occupational role and privileges. Professions restrict access to professional status and rewards through establishing entry gates, notably examinations and qualifications, which lead to the right to be listed on a professional register. Such a process may require legislation. Professionalization is a process whereby occupations seek recognition as an occupation that has specialized expertise requiring prolonged training, warranting the status of a profession. The boundaries between different occupations'/professions' areas of expertise and activity (such as care of normal childbirth and treatment of minor injuries) change over time and often require state legitimation. The creation and defence of socially constructed boundaries are seen as part of a 'professional project' (Larson 1977, Parkin 1979). Witz (1992) used the term 'professional project' to describe a process of collective action to gain/increase professional status through occupational demarcation via exclusion and usurpation. In health care she saw such strategies as competitive and conflictual, enacted within a hierarchical and patriarchal division of labour dominated by medicine. For subordinate groups like nursing and midwifery, taking on work traditionally the preserve of more powerful professions such as medicine (usurpation) can enhance professional status. Nevertheless, subordinate professions may need to adopt 'dual closure' strategies to ensure that other workers (such as support workers) are excluded from work activities that bring professional status and rewards. Health visitors, for example, are described in Part I as protective of their own role in parenting skills, and resentful of new groups of workers taking on such tasks. Boundary changes can increase, but also reduce, power.

Studies of changing professional boundaries have illustrated the prevalence of conflictual relationships between occupational groups at times of change. Timmons and Tanner (2004), for example, report on conflict between theatre nurses and operating department practitioners (ODPs), after ODPs secured professional status through the NHS Executive recognition of the voluntary register run by the Association of ODPs. In 2001 the NHS Executive issued guidance requiring all NHS Trusts to employ only ODPs on the register. Historically nurses were the dominant non-medical professional group working in operating theatres. Operating department practitioners did not have professional status so could not take on management roles within the operating department. Such roles were the preserve of nurses. Timmons and Tanner found considerable friction between a group of nurses and ODPs with nurses denigrating ODPs and emphasizing the importance of differences between the two groups, perceived as divides around the use of technology, providing support for doctors (ODPs) versus caring for patients (nurses) and the relative professional status of the two groups. Despite the recognition conferred by registration, nurses did not perceive ODPs as being members of a 'proper profession'. Although Timmons and Tanner suggest such open antagonism over demarcation issues is rare, Borthwick (2000) has recorded conflictual relationships between podiatric and orthopaedic surgeons, and Stevens *et al.* (2007) report on a lack of agreement about professional boundaries among eye-care professionals in the Netherlands. In a study of professional perspectives of ophthalmologists, GPs, optometrists and opticians, Stevens *et al.* found that whereas medical professionals were more likely to emphasize collective rather than idiosyncratic expertise, optometrists and opticians perceived expertise more often as an individual attribute. Ophthalmologists considered their expertise to be exclusive and their professional organization was strongly opposed to legislation in 2000 that gave Dutch optometrists the status of autonomous practitioner. Optometrists who claimed collective as well as idiosyncratic expertise reported doing more examinations, making more diagnoses, treating more and referring less than those who perceived expertise as an individual attribute. Hence commitment to a collective professionalizing project was related to levels of professional activity. The rise of optometrists, however, was accompanied by the declining status of opticians, who did not gain professional status. The study suggests that although shared care models across the groups are in progress, 'the competitive, exclusionary basis of professionalism seems to remain unchanged', with potentially negative consequences for collaboration. Nevertheless, whilst acknowledging the potential for conflict, Nancarrow and Borthwick (2005) have suggested that a consensual approach to boundary change is increasing. They note the significance of boundary change *within* professions as well as across professional groups and identify four directions of boundary change: diversification and specialization are intraprofessional processes; horizontal and vertical substitution occur across professions.

ACTIVITY

Note down any conflicts you have observed or experienced around role boundary changes in your own area of work. Consider the relevance of the four directions of boundary change.

These four directions of boundary change are illustrated in Part I. Intraprofessional processes are illustrated by the diversity of medicine and its range of specialities is represented through the voices of a GP, an emergency care consultant (ECC), a senior registrar in paediatrics (SRP), a consultant geriatrician, obstetric consultants and an obstetric registrar, and a psychiatrist. Nursing's increasing diversity and specialization (albeit more informal in organization than medical specialization) are reflected in the voices of different mental health nurses specializing in forensic mental health and in eating disorders, as well as a community nurse working in an intermediate home care team and adult nurses working in emergency care and in a respiratory specialism. The range of specialisms (both within and across professions) involved in acute care for children is illustrated by the children's nurse's comments when describing the multidisciplinary team in Chapter 2:

you have key nurses, hopefully you have the pain management team, the play specialist team, the occupational therapist team, the physiotherapist team, and then you've got clinical neurophysiologist coming in, the speech therapist coming in and the swallow team coming in . . . and then you have the schoolteachers . . .

Vertical substitution, as boundary change across professions, is illustrated by the devolution of specialized techniques such as ventouse delivery from doctors to midwives (see Chapter 4). Medical staff also devolved work to allied health professionals through health visitors carrying out immunizations, practice nurses taking cervical smears and conducting telephone triage for patients phoning about minor injuries and physiotherapists developing an independent role in management of knee injuries in A&E, which included taking responsibility for requesting X-rays. The ECC and SRP both expressed strong support for such vertical substitution. The SRP:

doctors can be great at doing many things, but there's quite a lot of stuff that anybody could do, so they're making a whole load of new roles now; so traditionally if someone is injured or did something to themselves, they'd come to hospital and a doctor would see them and patch them up; but now you have emergency care practitioners who used to be ambulance drivers...I like the change and I think that it frees up doctors to do different things.

Devolving tasks to support workers is also a key feature of workforce change. Support workers are referred to throughout Part I and such workers are receiving more and different training. Support workers in an intermediate home care team, discussed by Community nurse in Chapter 1, illustrate both horizontal and vertical substitution as they are 'physio-assistant and OT-assistant trained' as well as trained in 'basic personal care'. Hence the support workers 'as well as doing the basic personal care . . . they also do follow-up with the therapists . . . follow up exercises'. Such horizontal substitution is also practised by the professional staff, with nurses following a therapy programme 'that needs doing on a day that a nurse visit is planned . . . rather than sending in two or three different people'. Such flexibility and interprofessional co-operation benefit the service users by reducing the number of professionals involved and promoting continuity of care.

ACTIVITY

Note down any positive effects of role boundary changes in your work area from the point of view of professional staff, support workers, service managers and service users. Choose one example and identify aspects of staff behaviour that support a successful role change. Do you agree about the importance of flexibility and co-operation? Identify benefits, if any, for service users.

Policy initiatives have also encouraged horizontal and vertical substitution across lay and professional boundaries and across state and voluntary sectors. In Chapter 3 Service user(1) discusses her experience of the direct payment system, through which she is able to organize her own services. This involves taking on responsibility for employing staff so 'is not all plain sailing'. The government's Sure Start initiative led to closer working between health and social care professionals, voluntary agencies and local communities. In Chapter 3, a manager in a large voluntary agency described how the management board of the Sure Start local programme

> created posts like family support workers, midwife assistants and speech and language assistants, as well as volunteer posts such as Breastfeeding Babes supporters.

Despite successes, the support worker roles raised difficulties for some professions, such as speech and language therapy, as the professionals had to learn how to work in a different way, taking a community-wide view rather than a client perspective. The health visitor in Chapter 3 notes that the emphasis on voluntary sector and community support for parenting skills has challenged health visitors who 'thought that parenting was part of their remit'. Thus horizontal substitution across sector and lay/professional boundaries can lead to difficulties for established professionals. The established professionals are often expected to use their professional skills through a management rather than a case worker role, a change not welcomed by all. Nevertheless, Lord Darzi, leading the NHS *Next Stage Review*, himself a clinician, has strongly emphasized the importance of professionals with direct experience and responsibility for care being involved in managing change. His strategy for raising quality gives a central role to the empowerment of frontline staff, helping them 'innovate and improve the services they offer' (DH 2008:53–4), thus redressing the declining influence of clinicians in service management. It is these policies and patterns of workforce change that have led to an increased emphasis on the need to develop skills in leading interprofessional teams.

New skills for new services

Education for many professionals will now include leadership and management as part of pre- and post-qualifying curricula. The final report of the NHS *Next Stage Review* claims that in future every clinician will have the opportunity to be a practitioner, partner and leader. Darzi sees the acknowledgement of the importance of partnership in care, with collective accountability for performance, and the recognition of the importance of leadership at a variety of levels as constituting a new professionalism (DH 2008). At pre-qualifying level, however, leadership and management education has hitherto focused on managing within a uniprofessional team and its support staff. Voices in Part I illuminate the difficulties leading and managing interprofessional teams can create when professional staff are inadequately prepared for such roles.

OT(1)'s account of working in an integrated team for people with learning difficulties illustrate the challenges of managing integrated teams. OT(1) observes the challenges facing the team's manager:

> he's managed one profession but we're not one profession, we're lots of different professions, with all different standards and all different rates of pay and working hours and conditions . . .

The ECC is particularly clear about the management role of the consultant in the department, noting

> I often tell the juniors that one of the key skills about being a consultant is not about delivering good clinical care when you are there, it is about delivering good clinical care when you are not there. It is about setting up systems that facilitate high quality management . . . what you have to do is delegate.

He delegates work to the interprofessional team, not just to medical personnel. As such he exemplifies Darzi's vision of the role of clinicians in ensuring quality. As a practitioner he recognizes his accountability for the whole patient pathway and perceives himself as practitioner, partner and leader.

New ways of organising services, involving role redesign and closer partnerships between agencies, require new skills, particularly skills associated with teamworking. OT(1) identifies the importance of negotiation in managing role overlaps and reports that the experience of working together in the learning disabilities service has led to a change in thinking about team meetings – 'people are actually now thinking . . . how can you involve other people and help them feel more comfortable?' Teamworking involves thinking about the needs of team members. In Chapter 1 the GP recognizes that for doctors 'to survive in medical teams you have to value every member of that team for what they have to offer'. She sees it as essential that doctors should 'be trained that they are part of an interdisciplinary team, and the sooner medical students are introduced to that idea the better'. The ECC attributes the success of teamwork in emergency care settings to the lack of ingrained hierarchy due to the relative newness of the medical speciality. Hence

> the expectation of those being trained in the speciality is not that they are going to be called 'Sir' and wear a white coat and [be] followed around by a long trail of juniors.

He stresses the importance of communication and 'team ethos and atmosphere'. Reliance on hierarchy 'doesn't work'. Teamwork in modernized services involves open, democratic communication. Nevertheless the ECC trains medical staff for a leadership role:

> They do have to develop their skills and make decisions so the negotiation skills in terms of getting what you want in a way that is acceptable . . . it really hones people.

The ECC's account of his work illustrates the complexity of teamwork in current health and social care services. Professionals work in different types of teams. Some teams may be well established, with colleagues working together over many years. Some long-established teams will be hierarchically organised and well-functioning, others will be hierarchical and dysfunctional, as is illustrated in Chapter 5 for forensic psychiatry. In contrast, other teams will be time-limited. Pre-hospital emergency care, for example, requires collaboration in complicated, uncontrolled conditions.

> You are with people you have never met before and have to form teams in a very short space of time . . . How do you make teams work? How do you get things done effectively in a way that allows everyone to contribute?
>
> ECC, Chapter 2

These questions illustrate the importance of thinking, under pressure of time constraints, about effective ways of collaborating alongside effective use of professional knowledge.

―――――――――――――――――――― **ACTIVITY** ――――――――――――――――――――

Consider the teams you have worked in and how well they worked.

Focus on any examples of well-functioning teams and identify the skills of their members. How would you describe the teams? Were they established teams, time-limited teams, or integrated teams? It may help if you keep a diary of your collaborative work in teams over the course of a week. Reflect on the skills necessary in different types of teams.

Changing boundaries and interprofessional collaboration

Interprofessional vertical and horizontal substitution involve boundary changes that may present different challenges, exemplified in different types of teams. Horizontal substitution seems to be a common and necessary feature of integrated teams. Nies (2004:18) defines integrated care as ' a well-planned and well-organised set of services and care processes, targeted at the multidimensional needs/problems of an individual client, or a category of persons with similar needs/problems'. Integrated care, therefore, requires care provided through integrated processes that overcome professional and organizational barriers. In care of older people, for example, as Triantafillou (2004:113) explains, 'integrated teams aim to address the gaps in care for older people with complex health and social care needs that can occur between traditional services. They achieve this by offering a comprehensive and seamless care service', organized around the needs of the older person.

Whereas 'extracting' team members from their individual professional group is a main barrier to integrated teamwork, shared records, willingness to work flexibly, small teams, 'lowering' of professional roles (through acceptance of each other as equal co-professionals), accepting different ideas of leadership (according to the nature of the problem), exchanging staff between organizations and demonstrating effectiveness are all identified as factors supporting effective integrated teamworking (Triantafillou 2004).

Teamwork skills in integrated teams are complemented at an organizational level by the skills of 'boundary spanners' (Williams 2002:103). Boundary spanners are 'key agents managing within interorganisational theatres' (*ibid.*). The community development worker in Chapter 3, for example, reports that to improve services and facilities in a locality, 'we're often working in big partnership groups often across the whole of [county]'. Williams's research into the competencies of boundary spanners identified particular skills, abilities, experience and personal characteristics as:

- building sustainable relationships (through communicating and listening, understanding, empathizing, resolving conflict, demonstrating respect, honesty, openness, tolerance, approachability, building trust),

- managing through influencing and negotiation (networking is the *modus operandi* of choice),

- managing complexity and interdependencies through interorganizational experience, transdisciplinarity and cognitive capability,

- managing roles, accountabilities and motivations.

Many of these abilities have been identified as important in interprofessional working at many levels. The importance of interpersonal skills, essential for building sustainable relationships, is identified in the Interprofessional Capability Framework developed by a collaboration across universities supported by the Department of Health (Walsh *et al.* 2005) and confirmed in research into professionals' views of the skills required for interprofessional working (Pollard *et al.* 2008:49–58).

Vertical substitution is likely to take place within teams with a history of hierarchy, particularly a hierarchical structure dominated by the medical profession. Whereas such circumstances could lead to conflictual relationships, as already described, the literature suggests that hierarchical health care teams have often developed an effective way of working together, even if this has not been based on open communication. Relationships between doctors and nurses are particularly important in health care teams. Nurses have traditionally been expected to act on doctors' orders but exerted influence through what Stein (1967) described as a 'doctor–nurse game', a communication process whereby nurses made suggestions which doctors subsequently portrayed as their own ideas. Such communication may now be more open. The SRP in Chapter 2 tells us that the better doctors, the more experienced doctors, will do as they're told – and so that way it functions. Nurses know what they want and they often tell us what to do, and we do it.

Nevertheless, obstetric consultant(2) in Chapter 4 is aware of the persistence of medical dominance and sees teaching junior doctors respect for midwives as independent professionals as part of the job:

> we occasionally get the odd problem with a newish junior doctor, often male, [laughs] who insists on treating the midwives as nurses to do exactly as he tells them.

Ethnographic work in health care settings has confirmed that informal boundary blurring between medicine and nursing has been prevalent for many years. Hughes, in 1988, confirmed that nurses often worked in similar ways to doctors in A&E settings and Allen (1997) observed '*de facto* boundary blurring' between doctors and nurses even although they formally asserted separate jurisdiction. Hence formalizing nurses' role expansion into medical territory through, for example, undertaking endoscopy, ultrasound or breast examination may be building on a long tradition of collaborative informal role extension. Carmel (2006) has observed that the occupational boundary between doctors and nurses is obscured in an intensive care unit (ICU), 'whereas the organisational boundary (ICU–rest of hospital) is reinforced'. This suggests that in settings where professions work together in a shared space (such as A&E, obstetric units) for the benefit of a shared group of clients, flexible interprofessional teamwork can flourish, enabling vertical substitution. Carmel describes medicine and nursing as being incorporated into a joint ICU project. Doctors and nurses jointly established ICU outreach teams in which nurses took on aspects of medical work, gaining increased autonomy. This enhanced role for ICU nurses did not constitute a threat to consultants' authority as, on the contrary, ICU consultants could increase their own sphere of interest in the hospital. This interprofessional teamwork is described as 'an exemplary case of workplace empire building' and can be seen as an exemplary case of consensual vertical substitution. It is unclear, however, how the power of ICU as an organizational unit and interprofessional team affects the collaborative relationships with other hospital teams. Vertical substitution in settings which lack such organizational cohesion (such as nurse prescribing) may bring more uncertainty and may not be so consensual.

ACTIVITY

Consider your interprofessional collaboration in relation to your work setting and relationships. Do you work within an organizational unit or across organizations? Do you work differently with other professionals in different organizational settings? It may help if you keep a diary of your collaborative work over the course of a week. Reflect on your approaches to collaboration in different settings.

New models of professionalism

Whether or not changes in professional boundaries leads to uncertainty and to conflict is likely to depend on prevalent models of profession and professionalism. As Jones and Green (2006:928) note, 'in everyday discourse, references to "professionalism" are commonplace as distinguishers of preferred modes of occupational behaviour; claims to moral adequacy and markers of the limits to appropriate relationships with clients'. In recent years there has been considerable debate about professionals' claims to moral adequacy and appropriate modes of governance of professionals as well as debates about the relationship between professionals and the clients with whom they work. Changes in professional boundaries and professional claims to specialized expertise have accompanied such changes in discourse about professionalism. As early as 1995 Davies argued for a new model of professionalism to replace the 'old' notions of professionalism that she saw as grounded in patriarchy and cultural constructions of masculinity which emphasized the importance of autonomous practice. Davies's new model emphasized the importance of interdependent decision-making (involving clients and colleagues), reflective practice, collective responsibility and engagement rather than detachment. The model of professionalism advocated by Lord Darzi (DH 2008) reflects Davies's proposals. Accountability for services means health professionals must be partners as well as practitioners. Given that medicine remains the dominant profession in health care, it is interesting to explore possible changes in doctors' perceptions. Recent studies of medical practitioners have identified varied understandings of professionalism. In their study of GPs, Jones and Green (2006) found that early career GPs rejected a model of professionalism based on the notion of 'vocation' but also rejected 'old-fashioned' paternalism in relationships with clients, demonstrating a 'more democratic orientation towards both colleagues and patients' (p948). In contrast, Sanders and Harrison (2008), in a study of heart failure care, found that professionals involved in care employed four discourses as a means of establishing professional legitimacy: specialized expertise, competence, organizational efficiency and patient-centredness. Cardiologists relied solely on their specialized expertise, thus confirming their confident acceptance of 'the high status generally awarded to medical specialities that focus on acute conditions' (*ibid*.:304). Geriatricians adopted discourses of specialism, competence and patient-centredness, whereas GPs relied on competence and patient-centredness. Heart failure specialist nurses, however, utilized all four discourses, claiming expertise, competency, patient-centredness and organizational efficiency. Sanders and Harrison perceive the discursive field surrounding heart failure care as an arena for potential conflict, although they found no evidence of overt conflict. They argue that workforce change will lead professionals to adopt varied discursive strategies to redefine their roles and identities, as part of Lupton's (1997) process of reprofessionalization.

It is perhaps surprising that the specialist heart failure nurses did not claim teamworking or team co-ordination alongside organizational efficiency as a source of legitimacy. In the new NHS cardiologists relying on specialized expertise for their position in the health care team may find that their practitioner skills are insufficient for a lead role. Skills of partnership and leadership are also needed. D'Amour and Oandasan (2005), writing about health care, have proposed the concept of interprofessionality as providing a new frame of reference to understand cohesive practice amongst professionals from different disciplines. They argue that 'interprofessionality requires a paradigm shift since interprofessional practice has unique characteristics in terms of values, codes of conduct and ways of working' (*ibid.*:p9). These characteristics are:

- Patients are at the centre of collaborative care. This means their needs determine the interactions between professionals and they are able to participate in planning and delivering care.

- Professionals share common goals and have trusting personal and professional relationships. For such interaction to be possible, professionals need to be 'familiar with each others' conceptual models, roles and responsibilities'.

- Organisational factors such as leadership, governance and operating structures and systems all need to support interprofessional collaboration. (*ibid.*:15–17)

D'Amour and Oandasan note that our knowledge base about the processes involved in interprofessionality remain limited and must be developed. Development of such knowledge is likely to be crucial for health and social services to be able to deliver high quality care for all.

Summary

The materials and chapters in this book help to explore the complexity of interprofessional working. This chapter has reviewed traditional models of professionalism alongside changes in professional boundaries and working practices. The chapter notes that changes in role boundaries can be resisted through professional rivalry, insecurity, fears about losing areas of activity that bring job satisfaction, fears that skills are lost and services are inferior and fears of loss of power and status. On the other hand, flexibility around boundaries can benefit service users through promoting continuity of care, effective teamwork and through releasing time for highly trained staff to take on new skills and activities. Health and social care are delivered through different types of teams, with flexibility around professional boundaries being particularly important in integrated teams. There is a long history of successful collaboration across doctor–nurse boundaries in established teams in specific settings, but contemporary service delivery requires professionals to work collaboratively across varied and changing settings. Service development is underpinned by new models of professionalism and interprofessionalism. Successful interprofessional working involves both professionalism grounded in specialized skills and knowledge and in notions of service *and* interprofessionality.

References

Abbott A (1988) *The System of Professions: A Study of the Division of Expert Labour.* London:University of Chicago Press.

Allen D (1997) The nursing–medical boundary: a negotiated order? *Sociology of Health and Illness* 19(4):498–520.

Borthwick AM (2000) Challenging medicine: the case of podiatric surgery. *Work, Employment and Society* 14(2):369–83.

Carmel S (2006) Boundaries obscured and boundaries reinforced: incorporation as a strategy of occupational enhancement for intensive care. *Sociology of Health and Illness* 28(2):154–77.

D'Amour D, Oandasan I (2005) Interprofessionality as the field of interprofessional practice and education: an emerging concept. *Journal of Interprofessional Care* Supplement 1:8–20.

Davies C (1995) *Gender and the Professional Predicament in Nursing.* Buckingham:Open University Press.

DH (2008) *High Quality Care for All: NHS Next Stage Review Final Report.* Chair, Lord Darzi. CM 7432. London:The Stationery Office.

Dingwall R (1983) 'In the beginning was the work . . . .': reflections on the genesis of occupations. *Sociological Review* 31(4):605–24.

Finch J (2000) Interprofessional education and teamworking: a view from education providers. *British Medical Journal* 321:1138–40.

Freidson E (1970) *Profession of Medicine: A Study of the Sociology of Applied Knowledge.* Chicago:University of Chicago Press.

Harrison S (2002) New labour, modernisation and the medical process. *Journal of Social Policy* 31:465–85.

Haug MR (1973) Deprofessionalisation: an alternative hypothesis for the future. *Sociological Review* Monograph:195–212.

Hughes D (1988) When nurse knows best: some aspects of nurse/doctor interaction in a casualty department. *Sociology of Health and Illness* 10(1):1–21.

Jones L, Green J (2006) Shifting discourses of professionalism: a case study of general practitioners in the United Kingdom. *Sociology of Health and Illness* 28(7):927–50.

Larson MS (1977) *The Rise of Professionalism: A Sociological Analysis.* Berkeley:University of California Press.

Lupton D (1997) Doctors on the medical profession. *Sociology of Health and Illness* 19:480–97.

McKinlay JB, Stoekle JD (1988) Corporatization and the social transformation of doctoring. *International Journal of Health Services* 18(2):141–51.

Nancarrow SA, Borthwick AM (2005) Dynamic professional boundaries in the health care workforce. *Sociology of Health and Illness* 27(7):897–919.

Nies H (2004) Integrated care: concepts and background. In: Nies H, Berman PC (eds) *Integrating Services for Older People: A resource book for managers.* Dublin:European Health Management Association,17–31.

Parkin F (1979) *Marxism and Class Theory: A Bourgeois Critique.* London:Tavistock.

Pollard K, Rickaby C, Miers M (2008) *Evaluating student learning in an interprofessional curriculum: the relevance of pre-qualifying interprofessional education for future professional practice.* HEA Health Science and Practice Subject Centre with UWE, Bristol. www.health.heacademy. ac.uk/projects/miniprojects/completeproj.htm

Sanders T, Harrison S (2008) Professional legitimacy claims in the multidisciplinary workplace: the case of heart failure care. *Sociology of Health and Illness* 30(2):289–308.

Stein L (1967) The doctor–nurse game. *Archives of General Psychiatry* 16:699–703.

Stevens FCJ, Diederiks JPM, Grit F, van der Horst F (2007) Exclusive, idiosyncratic and collective expertise in the interprofessional arena: the case of optometry and eye care in the Netherlands. *Sociology of Health and Illness* 29(4):481–96.

Timmons S, Tanner J (2004) A disputed occupational boundary: operating theatre nurses and Operating Department Practitioners. *Sociology of Health and Illness* 26(5):645–66.

Triantafillou J (2004) Integrated teams. In: Nies H, Berman PC (eds) *Integrating Services for Older People: A Resource Book for Managers.* Dublin:European Health Management Association,113–28.

Walsh CL, Gordon MF, Marshall M, Wilson F, Hunt T (2005) Interprofessional capability: a developing framework for interprofessional education. *Nurse Education in Practice* 5:230–7.

Williams P (2002) The competent boundary spanner. *Public Administration* 80:115–127.

Witz A (1992) *Professions and Patriarchy.* London:Routledge.

The Medicalization Thesis

Katherine C Pollard

Introduction

Interprofessional interaction in health and social care is primarily a social activity involving ways of understanding and communicating which have resulted from both occupational and wider social conditioning. So in order to understand interprofessional working in health and social care, we should also examine it in relation to the wider social context. Many theorists argue that modern Western society is markedly *medicalized*, in that the medical perspective is normatively applied to social phenomena (Nettleton 2006). This argument is known as 'the medicalization thesis'. In this chapter, interprofessional working in health and social care will be examined in relation to the medicalization thesis.

The evolution of medicalization

During the age of enlightenment, the application of the scientific approach to physical phenomena resulted in its becoming the dominant paradigm in Western society (Smith 1998). Areas of scientific enquiry included anatomy and physiology. Medical practitioners incorporated this new knowledge into their curative practices, and medicine accordingly developed into a scientific discipline. The rise of professionalism also strengthened medical practitioners' social standing and ambit (Witz 1992). The history of medicine over the last two centuries shows how doctors defined and delineated their profession and their sphere of practice; and, importantly, how they successfully lobbied state institutions to secure a powerful social position (Nettleton 2006).

In the 1960s, social theorists started to write about 'the medicalisation thesis' (Nye 2003). In this context, 'medicalization' means the application of the medical model to social activities. A key feature of the medical model is the belief that health, with a few exceptions, is dependent on internal physiological factors (rather than on social or environmental conditions) (Nettleton 2006). Medicalization of a social situation, therefore, implies that social problems arise due to individuals' behaviour and/or circumstances, rather than being caused by wider factors. Medicalization can therefore result in individuals' behaviour being categorized as 'deviant' or 'pathological' if it departs from standards laid down by the medical profession:

> Medical models have influenced standards of pathology and norm, therapeutic philosophies and techniques, strategies for social intervention, and theories of deviance and punishment. Where they have gained ascendance, such models have historically threatened, and occasionally supplanted, civil and human rights in modern states.
>
> Nye (2003:115)

Such a situation obviously involves the operation of power – but how does any particular perspective become dominant in a society? Underlying the medicalization thesis is the argument that knowledge is socially constructed, rather than being indisputable 'fact' (which is often the scientific view). For social constructionists, all knowledge is value-laden, in that it is mediated through individuals' internal mental and emotional processes (Smith 1998, Nettleton 2006).

One of the first theorists to write about medicalization was Michael Foucault. He linked theories of power and knowledge to explain the pervasiveness of the medical model in Western society (Foucault 1973). Foucault argued that the exercise of power involves using knowledge to structure and fix what is considered 'normal'. So for example, in the nineteenth and early twentieth centuries, doctors used their claim to exclusive, scientific knowledge to enhance their social influence. As they were increasingly regarded as the authorities on health and disease, their sphere of influence and practice grew, medical knowledge was increasingly privileged, and the medical viewpoint became normalized in many areas of life (Nettleton 2006, Helman 2007). Other viewpoints, such as that of social care, in which a social, rather than medical, model of health and wellbeing is adopted, were consequently held to be relatively unimportant.

Illich (1984:161) spoke about 'cultural iatrogenesis' to describe the condition in which natural 'healthy' acceptance of sickness and death is suppressed. He felt that, when 'health management designed on the engineering model' is adopted within a society, 'better health' is viewed as a commodity. The belief that doctors can provide this commodity results in medicalization. To appreciate the extent to which Western society is medicalized, it is useful to contrast it with societies in which other beliefs prevail. For example, mental health problems in some societies are considered primarily to involve spiritual dimensions, being therefore the domain of spiritual healers, rather than of medical practitioners (Helman 2007). Consideration of the effects of medicalization should therefore incorporate acknowledgement that any social phenomenon can be approached from a number of perspectives.

===== **ACTIVITY** =====

Consider a situation where an individual is physically healthy, but finding it difficult to cope with life emotionally and mentally. Who do you think is the best person to support this individual? Try and decide why you have chosen this person – is it because of their knowledge, their skills, their personality, their occupation, or some other reason?

An illustration of how medical knowledge is applied to social situations in our own society is evident in the way that unruly children are frequently diagnosed with attention deficit disorder. In this way, an essentially social situation is framed as being intrinsically a medical issue (Nye 2003). The consequence is that these children are commonly medicated, rather than offered other forms of interaction or activity which might help them to develop socially acceptable behaviour. In 2005 nearly 400,000 children in the UK were medicated for this purpose (Ragg 2006). Similarly, 'shyness' is sometimes perceived as a pathological condition, which can be treated using various strategies, including medication (Nye 2003, Scott 2006).

It is interesting to note that there was explicit mention in Part I of specific social situations and activities with an accompanying assumption that health care professionals would (should?) be involved in them:

It might be that they've suffered a bereavement . . . it's something that maybe a CPN [Community Psychiatric Nurse] could help with.

Community nurse, Chapter 1

if . . . there's an older child . . . and there's problems there, mother's not really knowing about play, what the best things are to do . . . I'll tell the mother 'would it be ok with you if the playworker comes along, just to talk through that?'

Health visitor, Chapter 1

they [health visitors] are supposed to concentrate on children in need and have an increased role around parenting skills.

Manager of large voluntary agency (MLVA), Chapter 3

Bereavement, play and parenting are inherently *social* activities/issues: in many societies, they are not automatically assumed to be areas requiring input, either directly or indirectly, from health professionals. Although non-medical health care professionals may not consider themselves to be allied with a specifically medical viewpoint, it should be remembered that many modern health-care professions, particularly nursing and midwifery, have been developed and regulated in accordance with medical perceptions of illness and risk (Witz 1992, Leap 2004, Pollard 2007). It can therefore be argued that these quotes are indicative of the high level of medicalization in the UK today.

It should also be noted that the medical perspective is often linked with the moral high ground (Riska 2003). There is an expectation that 'good citizens' will follow medical advice about healthy living. In this way, the medical perspective on what constitutes a 'correct' lifestyle has become internalized within the population (Nye 2003). It is also increasingly reinforced through legislation, as evidenced by the ban on smoking instituted in various Western countries over since the late 1990s.

================================= **ACTIVITY** =================================

Consider a situation where someone has been prescribed medication for a particular condition, but has decided not to take it. What is your opinion of this course of action? Try and see what ideas and assumptions your opinion is based on. Who do you think should have final say about how people behave with regard to their own health? Why?

Gender issues

Medicalization cannot be discussed without considering gender issues. The notion of gender is culturally determined, and has been assigned various attributes in different times and different societies: in the Western world, these attributes were traditionally conceptualized as binary opposites, for example, masculine/feminine and strong/weak (Annandale 1998). Moreover, 'masculine' attributes were generally assigned positive social value, while many 'feminine' attributes were distrusted as socially aberrant and leading to behaviour requiring male control (Annandale 1998, Nye 2003). These binary conceptions have been challenged and, to some extent, overturned over the last century (Annandale 1998). However, during the nineteenth century, the rise of medicine as a rational, 'masculine' science resulted in the irrational and the 'feminine' becoming pathologized, and the effects of this are still discernible.

One of the most obvious targets for medicalization has been women's health. In very many countries, legislation gives medical practitioners power over women giving birth. Pregnancy is therefore equated with illness, in that it is seen as requiring surveillance and management by medically oriented health professionals to be brought to a safe and healthy conclusion (Nettleton 2006). Similarly, the normal physiological process of menopause has been defined as an 'endocrine deficiency' with accompanying 'symptoms', widely treated through pharmaceutical means (Helman 2007). Medicalization can therefore itself be considered a gendered process (Riska 2003).

A relatively recent phenomenon affecting gendered notions and processes inherent in medicalization is the feminization of the workplace. In this context, 'feminization' implies not only a greater proportion of the workforce being female than previously; but also the way in which issues of self-presentation and image at work now apply both to male and female employees (Adkins 2002). Relatively informal modes of dress and communication are increasingly common, and there is growing recognition of the need for 'emotional intelligence' at work, that is, for individuals to be aware of their own and other people's emotions and sensitivities (Rutherford 2001, Adkins 2002). An associated aspect of feminization is the increasing privileging of what was formerly seen as essentially a female tendency, that is, the trend for individuals to make sense of their occupational roles through interpersonal communication and relationships, and to take opportunities to 'be themselves' at work (Rutherford 2001, Erickson and Pierce 2005).

However, feminization does not imply a shift in power either from men to women, or from traditionally 'masculine' to traditionally 'feminine' roles and occupations (Riska 2001, Erickson and Pierce 2005). Whatever the developments in the wider social sphere, the process of feminization appears to have made little substantive impact on power and influence within health or social care professions. For example, men in nursing and social work, despite their relatively small numbers, are disproportionately over-represented at senior levels in these professions (Whittock *et al*. 2002, Christie 2006). Conversely, although there are many women doctors, they are over-represented in medical specialities which are comparatively poorly paid and of low status within the profession (Riska 2001).

Technology

Another feature of contemporary life linked with medicalization is technology. Modern medicine's efficacy depends heavily on technological equipment and techniques, for example, ultrasound scanning and laparoscopic surgery. Medicine is therefore a prime site for technologization, which, in Western society, is associated with progress (Nettleton 2006). It is unsurprising, therefore, that increased medicalization of social activities is commonly viewed as being universally beneficial. The authority given to the scientific and technological paradigms, together with the historical professional dominance of medicine, ensures that the medical perspective continues to be privileged in our society.

Changes in the organization of health care

Despite the ongoing dominance of medicine *per se*, the overall picture in the UK is becoming increasingly complex. Since the late 1970s many non-medical health professions have been engaging in 'professionalization projects' in order to gain greater status, autonomy and influence in relation to each other, to the medical profession and to wider social structures (Annandale 1998, Nettleton 2006) (see Chapter 8). These projects can entail taking over areas of practice which doctors relinquish, willingly or unwillingly (Nancarrow and Borthwick 2005, Pollard 2007). This situation was acknowledged by the GP interviewed in Chapter 1:

> The way things have moved, there is a tranche of their [doctors'] work that can be done by other people and one of the most important things is, for doctors to survive they have to give away some of their work.

It is also important to recognize that the rise of a commercial ethos in health care, coupled with an emphasis on service users' rights, has effected radical change in the organization of medical institutions (Annandale 1998, Lissauer 2003). Even the illusion of autonomy and control is no longer available to many junior doctors, for example, owing to increasingly complex organizational structures, managerial demands, budgetary constraints and calls for public accountability. There is also currently an unprecedented move for greater regulation for doctors (GMC 2008).

In a bid to utilize the workforce more efficiently, many procedures and competencies previously monopolized by the medical profession have been opened up to other occupations. In this way, they have been redefined as being technically, rather than professionally, based; that is, occupation alone does not determine who may conduct them (Cameron and Masterson 2003). Doctors interviewed for Part II mentioned this:

> what the government's trying to do across health care . . . is look at what job needs doing, and see who's best able to do that – and there are different benefits, but I guess one is going to be a cost saving. So doctors can be great at doing many things, but there's quite a lot of stuff that they do that anybody could do.
>
> Senior registrar, paediatrics (SRP)

However, despite the apparent threat to its authority and influence, the medical profession still exerts considerable power at strategic levels. Economic factors dictate policy and procedures in most NHS Trusts in the UK; this includes adherence to evidence-based clinical practice, for fear of litigation (Samanta and Samanta 2004). The National Institute for Clinical Excellence (NICE) provides guidelines to clinicians to this end; however, these guidelines depend on who evaluates available research. Members of NICE committees and review panels are drawn mainly from the medical profession and NHS management (NICE 2007).

It can be argued that the privileging of medical knowledge, the persistence of gendered perspectives, the technological imperative and the dominance of the medical profession, as described above, have resulted in a significant degree of medicalization within the UK and many other Western societies. Of course, there may be many individuals, both members of the public and the professions, who would disagree with this argument. However, it can be argued that support for the medicalization thesis in academic circles and consideration of the points raised above constitute sufficient grounds for further exploration of this topic. In the next section of this chapter, interprofessional interaction and relationships within the context of a medicalized society are discussed.

Interprofessional working

Since the late 1970s, there has been growing recognition that satisfactory care delivery entails collaboration involving a range of workers, both professional and non-professional, across a number of sectors, including social care (WHO 1978, DH 2008). It appears that these developments have given the medical perspective legitimacy in its application to the wider social context. This argument is supported by the involvement of medically oriented health professionals in essentially social areas such as bereavement, children's play and parenting, as demonstrated above.

Examination of various aspects of interprofessional and inter-agency working can reveal wider effects of medicalization. In particular, it is useful to investigate whether/how the factors listed above are evident in interaction involving individuals from a range of occupations and backgrounds.

The privileging of medical knowledge

The privileging of medical knowledge is underpinned by the belief that the medical view about any issue is better than any other view. Looking at material drawn from Chapter 2, it appears that this belief can be expressed through a variety of forms:

> one of the problems we came across really early on was X-rays. A lot of people need X-rays . . . wherever possible we'd encourage the practitioners themselves to develop their own [training] programmes but they often need the medical rubber stamp.
>
> Emergency care consultant (ECC)

> have just started that we are allowed to write in the child's medical notes . . . the doctors are quite happy as long as we don't do nurse writing which is like reams.
>
> Children's nurse

These two quotes show that, not only must other practitioners' knowledge be ratified by the medical profession, but also that, if they are to be trusted to contribute to an individual's medical record, they must modify their style to suit the medical profession (in many NHS institutions, different occupational groups still use different paper records, in which only members of that particular occupation write).

This situation can, unsurprisingly, lead to conflict between non-medical health professionals and medical practitioners:

> I have never worked particularly closely with GPs . . . in [area], where they were single-handed most of the time, I was fighting against a lot of the advice they gave.
>
> Health visitor, Chapter 1

> some of the babies that they class as small for dates, as well, the paediatricians can be quite funny about them and they say, 'Oh, they've got to have two weight gains before they go home', and you say, 'Well, actually, they're feeding really well, they're weeing, they're pooing, they're pink and warm . . . the weight was only this', and you have to sort of be a bit forceful with them sometimes.
>
> Community midwife(3), Chapter 4

The material in Chapter 4 does, however, also appear to illustrate incidents of medical practitioners' acknowledging the value of other professionals' knowledge and/or skills:

> they're professionals in their own right . . . midwives are there to be the professional-looking after normal pregnancy, normal labour . . . midwives have their area of expertise.
>
> Obstetric consultant(2)

> most of the senior midwives are going to be a lot more experienced in their career than I ever will be at normal midwifery.
>
> Obstetric registrar

However, the impact of these statements is lessened when one considers that midwives' remit and professional body of knowledge concerning 'normality' in pregnancy and birth have been constructed by the medical profession, according to medically defined notions of risk (Leap 2004). Jowitt (2001) noted that NICE guidelines affecting midwifery practice are based on obstetric and paediatric principles and priorities, rather than on midwifery principles. So it appears that the medical perspective still implicitly prevails in this situation.

If other professionals' knowledge is assumed to be inferior to that of the medical profession, service users' knowledge appears to be given only very little, if any, value. When discussing the requirement that parents be referred to paediatricians should they not wish their newborn babies to receive a Vitamin K injection, a community midwife interviewed in Chapter 4 ranked sources of knowledge, assuming that medical knowledge was superior to midwifery knowledge, and that service users needed medical input in order for their knowledge to be adequate for the situation. She also illustrated the normalisation of medical knowledge, describing it as 'unbiased' knowledge:

> we have to try and give information in a very unbiased way, and with as much medical knowledge . . . as possible; . . . the parents don't always have the full information and

knowledge at their fingertips to make a decision, and so I do feel somebody even more in the know than me [the paediatricians] can still give them unbiased information.

Community midwife(1)

Similarly, the SRP described in Chapter 3 how a paediatric consultant related to patients only by telling them what she thought they needed to know:

she kept describing information she was giving, she wants the patient apparently to fit in with our agenda, on the basis that if you do as we tell you, you'll get better, so if you take your treatments properly, if you have this kind of diet, if you do these things.

This goes against the principle that service users should be considered as partners in care, and that the service user voice should be heard in the process of service provision (Thomas 2005).

Although the medicalization thesis criticizes the widespread medicalization of society, there is obviously no suggestion that medical knowledge is without value. A quote from a social worker in Chapter 5 illustrates how important medical input can be:

Now if I had been a lone worker . . . as we are in the disabled adults team . . . I would go out and you would recognise the difficulties. But you wouldn't necessarily pick up on what the consultant psychiatrist picked up on which was the medication. He'd [the service user] been prescribed medication that had interacted with other medications that he was prescribed and that was causing him to exhibit some of the behaviour that he was exhibiting . . . Now if I'd gone out on my own I wouldn't necessarily have been aware of this . . . and we could have masked the problem.

Social worker(3)

The argument is, however, that other forms of knowledge should also be acknowledged and used where appropriate – other individuals made it clear in Chapter 5 that the medical perspective is not necessarily always the best vantage point from which to view a situation:

[doctors] are only human at the end of the day. If they have travelled all that way they might be very good at rationally thinking things through in terms of medicine, but dealing with a whole group of people and thinking about medical matters at the same time, I think is inefficient.

Mental health nursing student(3)

it's very important for what we deliver that it is a multidisciplinary, multiprofessional way of working because in terms of thinking about eating disorders, there is no one way that works . . . psychologists or psychiatrists don't have the magic answer . . . you have to think all across the board and that's why we need people to bring all of their skills to what we do.

Mental health nurse(1)

they [psychiatrists] work within a medical framework so they, they're making a diagnosis of mental disorder, you know, they're prescribing treatments . . . I think everybody would agree that risk isn't just to do with a mental disorder, you know, you have to look at a lot of other things as well.

Psychologist

=================== **ACTIVITY** ===================

Think about who you consider to be really knowledgeable about different aspects of life. Who are these people? Can you rank them according to the knowledge they hold? What makes one person's knowledge more useful than another's? Try and see what ideas and assumptions underpin your answer to this question.

Gendered perspectives

The gendered nature of the medical perspective is evident in the way that health professionals do not prioritize issues that they feel are unimportant. When examined, these often include those traditionally within the remit of women, namely, emotional wellbeing and domestic concerns, as is shown by quotes from Chapter 4:

they weren't really explaining to me why it would be a great thing if I got induced, they were explaining to me why they were going to induce me essentially . . . it was almost like, 'You're ours now, we can do what we like and that's it, you're here', almost, rather than working with, you know, somebody who's clearly heavily pregnant, clearly quite upset.

Service user(3)

We went into the hospital that evening and they monitored us and tried to convince me to stay in, and I also have two small children at home, I wasn't keen on that . . . [the obstetric registrar] just wasn't communicative and wasn't able to understand that we might not be keen on . . . staying in hospital, he just seemed to think that whatever he suggested ought to be exactly what we did.

Service user(4)

There is also an assumption that women's behaviour in the social sphere is a legitimate area of concern for health care professionals, as in the example concerning the 'right' way to play with children (see above), although workers and professionals from non-health sectors may be involved:

The health visitor is the team leader, and there may be nursery nurses . . . health visitor assistants . . . playworkers . . . the health visitor won't necessarily have all the contacts with the family, but will have the overall remit for that family . . . [the health visitor is] the core, the main person, really.

Health visitor, Chapter 1

So this situation can be interpreted as a demonstration of how our society, the development of whose wider health care services have been heavily influenced by the medical viewpoint, sees the need to control women's behaviour for fear of 'aberrant' outcomes.

The gendered medical perspective also affects individuals working within the care services, most notably nurses. The organization of nursing in the UK in the late nineteenth and early twentieth centuries combined aspects of the military model with the perception that nurses were socially comparable to female domestic employees 'in service'; hence the wearing of uniforms and a hierarchical 'chain of command'. Traces of this gendered hierarchy can be seen in comments made by individuals quoted in Part II:

B team is consultant-led completely . . . The B team meeting . . . is very formal . . . nurses can have their say but it's intimidating, it's threatening.

Children's nurse, Chapter 2

There is a medical model here . . . there's one or two [consultant psychiatrists] who are very much the old school, you know, I snap my fingers and you as a nurse do what I say.

Nursing officer, Chapter 5

There can be little doubt that interprofessional relationships are influenced by these gendered structures and processes. Interestingly, the ECC in Chapter 2 thought that this situation would be improved by bringing more women into medicine:

I suspect that with increasing numbers of female doctors we will see increasingly better teamwork. We are a bit stuck in the 'male doctors–female nurses', underlying gender issues, there's a kind of hierarchy that seems to be perpetuated. But with increase in medical graduates being women . . . I expect that means we'll see better teamworking.

A female obstetrician in Chapter 4 was also of the opinion that it was usually male junior obstetricians who felt the need to assert their authority:

we occasionally get the odd problem with a newish junior doctor, often male, [laughs] who insists on treating the midwives as nurses to do exactly as he tells them.

Obstetric consultant(2)

However, the view that it is only men in the system who cause problems is rather simplistic. There is ample evidence that female health professionals both reinforce the gendered hierarchy and police their colleagues in order to maintain it (Robertson 2004).

If you are a health or social care professional, consider how colleagues behave when working across occupations/disciplines. Is there a difference between the behaviour of male and female colleagues? Is there a difference between the behaviour of colleagues from different disciplines? Try and decide whether or not any of these differences could be related to gender issues. Are there any other social factors that could be relevant here?

The technological imperative

It appears that doctors still defend their right to control technology which they consider to be their domain:

> There'll always be anxiety about allowing another [non-medical] profession to request an X-ray . . . although we have had a lot of success with this, even some of my colleagues have been persistently reluctant; 'Ooh I don't know about this', depending on their mindset.
>
> ECC, Chapter 2

Both obstetricians in Chapter 4 thought that midwife ventouse practitioners enjoyed enhanced status within the maternity services:

> I think people are just really pleased if they've got a midwife ventouse practitioner on with them, because they actually see that person as being much more their kind of key helper than, for example, the junior doctor who runs around, but can't actually get the women delivered.
>
> Obstetric consultant(2)

This emphasis on the desirability of technical and/or technological competence, inherent in the medical perspective, accordingly impacts on both boundaries between professions, and relationships between different professionals. In particular, those possessing skills only in non-technical areas, such as interpersonal skills and the provision of basic care, are often viewed as being of less value and usually have lower status in the organization (Pollard 2007).

Whatever your occupation, identify the people you most value, and those with the most valuable skills in your organization. Why have you chosen these individuals? Try and see what ideas and assumptions underpin your choice.

The dominance of the medical profession

Traditionally, the medical profession has controlled the practice of related professionals (Nettleton 2006). However, the degree to which individuals can participate in interprofessional working in a way which is meaningful to them is undoubtedly important. The concept of 'parity' has been invoked in this regard:

> Parity requires, and is fostered by, participation and involvement which ensures that people have some real say in decisions which affect their work.
>
> Meads and Ashcroft (2005:21)

It is interesting to note that, despite the continuing privileging of the medical perspective, professionals in Part I have reported developments in the organization of care delivery that promote wider participation in decision-making processes:

> When [interprofessional working] is working well, it's really successful . . . the physios are quite happy to come down and assess . . . originally . . . if we needed [patients] to be assessed . . . it would have to be a medical admission.
>
> Adult nurse(2), Chapter 2

Other changes in service delivery also appear to have altered the position of doctors as individuals (not always to their satisfaction) in relation to some other professionals:

> Nowadays midwives are much more independent practitioners than they used to be, linking much less with GPs. This is a point of contention as the GP's role is much less than it used to be.
>
> GP, Chapter 1

However, medical professionals still often have authority over other professions:

> The role of the consultant in an emergency department is to oversee the management of all the patients by all the staff . . . You are not necessarily always physically present, but you are still responsible for what goes on.
>
> ECC, Chapter 2

> I would imagine that most doctors work along a doctor agenda and everything revolves around them, they feel they're busy and important, so they will turn up on a ward round, they expect nurses to drop what they're doing to attend the ward round and support them.
>
> SRP, Chapter 2

There is a perception that this is not always appropriate in the interprofessional context:

> some consultants on the B side get very over-involved and try to dictate who is involved in the multidisciplinary team.
>
> Children's nurse, Chapter 2

> The better doctors, the more experienced doctors, will do as they're told . . . Nurses know what they want and they often tell us what to do, and we do it.
>
> SRP, Chapter 2

In the wider context, relationships between social care and health care professionals can often reflect conflicting values (Glasby and Littlechild 2004). In Chapter 3, the MLVA commented on the anomaly she perceived within DH guidelines about children's services:

> there was no mention of partnership or collaboration . . . It gave the strong view that they [health visitors] were the only leaders, the people who ran the show for early years.

However, there appears to be growing awareness that this is not a particularly constructive stance, and other health care professionals speaking in Part I reported a far more egalitarian approach to working with their social care colleagues:

> they're [social workers] not coming from a medical model and they're funded in a completely different way . . . when I've had dealings with social workers it's been very much a kind of mutual respect for each other's profession but they're quite distinct.
>
> Community midwife(2), Chapter 4

> the social workers are quite new to the medical side of things . . . the clinical meetings have actually changed to service users' meetings and lost the name of the clinical meetings to make [the social workers] feel more comfortable with it.
>
> Occupational therapist(1), Chapter 1

So it appears that the dominance of the medical profession is being challenged to some extent. However, there appears still to be a wider perception that doctors and other health professionals wield legitimate authority over other individuals:

> Before her husband died, they were receiving visits from home care assistants, and district nurses came three times a week, as her husband required regular medical input. Service user(1) described the district nurses as 'for want of a better word, very nosy – they can rule your life'.
>
> Service user(1), Chapter 3

The ambulance personnel are in charge of the medical response . . . The police and the fire service on the scene all just expect the doctor to be in charge of the medical response, but the ambulance service might subscribe to a different view.

ECC, Chapter 2

Nevertheless, it appears that, despite still enjoying a considerable degree of authority, individual medical practitioners are not quite so powerful as they once were, in that they no longer have the freedom to practise without taking into consideration issues of teamworking and other professionals' opinions and contributions (Nettleton 2006). However, there seems to have been little diminution in medicalization *per se* – medical knowledge is still privileged, gender is still an issue, and the technological imperative prevails. Interprofessional developments in health and social care, therefore, are necessarily framed within the wider social context in which medicalization is accepted and assumed to be 'normal'. So rather than negotiation between differing perspectives, interprofessional working in our society largely entails collaboration between different occupations sharing similar perceptions about health and wellbeing. Tensions that arise are then often due to disagreements as to whose concerns should be prioritized, rather than due to fundamental differences between individuals' understanding of the issues involved (Pollard 2007).

Summary

Interprofessional interaction in health and social care is primarily a social activity. In order to understand it fully, we should therefore also examine it with regard to the wider social context. This chapter has examined interprofessional working in relation to the medicalization thesis, which argues that the medical perspective is often inappropriately applied to a range of inherently social phenomena. This process can result in individuals' behaviour being considered deviant, should they go against medical advice concerning 'correct' lifestyles.

Key features of medicalization are:

- medical knowledge is privileged above other forms of knowledge,
- gendered perspectives promote medical control of women's health and behaviour,
- the technological imperative reinforces medical dominance,
- the medical profession exercises authority over related occupations and the wider public,
- medical models of wellbeing take precedence over social models.

Medicalization of society therefore influences interprofessional interaction and relationships, which are still dictated by the assumption that in most situations doctors know more, and are therefore deserving of higher status, than other individuals. Health professionals still operate to a large extent within a gendered hierarchy, and those with technological skills are considered to be more valuable than those equipped only with non-technological skills.

However, changes in the organization and ethos of care delivery, together with the wider feminization of the workplace, have resulted in challenges to the status of the medical profession: individual medical practitioners must now consider the opinions and contributions of other occupational groups and of service users. Nevertheless, the move towards greater collaboration within care delivery over the last 30 years has resulted in the medical perspective gaining greater legitimacy in its application to a range of social activities. The medical viewpoint therefore seems to have become increasingly dominant in our society. Consequently, from the vantage point of the medicalization thesis, it appears that interprofessional working often involves collaboration between professionals from different health and social care disciplines who largely agree in their perception of what healthy living entails, rather than negotiation between individuals/groups with fundamentally differing perspectives regarding these issues.

References

Adkins L (2002) *Revisions: Gender and Sexuality in Late Modernity.* Buckingham:Open University Press.

Annandale E (1998) *The Sociology of Health and Medicine: A Critical Introduction.* Cambridge:Polity Press.

Cameron A, Masterson A (2003) Reconfiguring the Clinical Workforce. In: Davies C (ed) *The Future Health Workforce.* Basingstoke:Palgrave Macmillan, 68–86.

Christie A (2006) Negotiating the uncomfortable intersections between gender and professional identities in social work. *Critical Social Policy* 26(2):390–411.

DH (2008) *NHS Next Stage Review: Our Vision for Primary and Community Care.* London: Department of Health.

Dingwall R, Rafferty AM, Webster C (1988) *An Introduction to the Social History of Nursing.* London:Routledge.

Erickson K, Pierce JL (2005) Farewell to the organization man: the feminization of loyalty in high-end and low-end service jobs. *Ethnography* 6(3):283–313.

Foucault M (1973) *The Birth of the Clinic: An Archaeology of Medical Perception.* London:Tavistock.

Glasby J, Littlechild R (2004) *The Health and Social Care Divide: The Experiences of Older People.* (rev. 2nd edn) Bristol:The Policy Press.

GMC (2008) *Licensing and Revalidation.* www.gmc-uk.org/about/reform/index.asp (Accessed 24.9.08).

Helman CG (2007) *Culture, Health and Illness.* (5th edn) New York:Hodder Arnold.

Illich I (1984) The epidemics of modern medicine. In: Black N, Boswell D, Gray A, Murphy S, Popay J (eds) *Health & Disease: A Reader.* Milton Keynes:Open University Press, 156–62.

Jowitt M (2001) Not very NICE: induction of labour draft guidelines – a commentary. *Midwifery Matters* 89:23–5.

Leap N (2004) Journey to midwifery through feminism: a personal account. In: Stewart M (ed) *Pregnancy, Birth and Maternity Care: Feminist Perspectives.* Edinburgh:Books for Midwives Press, 185–200.

Lissauer R (2003) Delivering a patient-centred service: reforming professional roles. In: Davies C (ed) *The Future Health Workforce*. Basingstoke:Palgrave Macmillan,14–32.

Meads G, Ashcroft J (2005) Policy into practice: collaboration. In: Meads G, Ashcroft J, with Barr H, Scott R, Wild A *The Case for Interprofessional Collaboration in Health and Social Care*. Oxford:Blackwell, 15–35.

Nancarrow SA, Borthwick AM (2005) Dynamic professional boundaries in the health care workforce. *Sociology of Health and Illness* 27(7):897–919.

Nettleton S (2006) *The Sociology of Health and Illness*. (2nd edn) Cambridge:Polity Press.

NICE (2007) *National Institute for Health and Clinical Excellence*. www.nice.org.uk (Accessed 8.01.2007).

Nye R (2003) The evolution of the concept of medicalization in the late twentieth century. *Journal of History of the Behavioural Sciences* 39(2):115–29.

Pollard K (2007) *Discourses of unity and division: a study of interprofessional working among midwives in an English NHS maternity unit*. PhD thesis, University of the West of England, Bristol.

Ragg R (2006) School uniformity. *Ecologist on-line* www.theecologist.org/archive_detail.asp?content_id=621 (Accessed 22.09.2006).

Riska E (2001) Towards gender balance: but will women physicians have an impact on medicine? *Social Science and Medicine* 52:179–87.

Riska E (2003) Gendering the medicalization thesis. *Advances in Gender Research* 7:59–87.

Robertson J (2004) Changing a culture of horizontal violence. *The Practising Midwife* 7(2):40–1.

Rutherford S (2001) Any difference? An analysis of gender and divisional management styles in a large airline. *Gender, Work and Organization* 8(3):326–34.

Samanta A, Samanta J (2004) NICE guidelines and law: clinical governance implications for trusts. *Clinical Governance: An International Journal* 9(4):212–15.

Scott S (2006) The medicalisation of shyness: from social misfits to social fitness. *Sociology of Health and Illness* 28(2):133–53.

Smith MJ (1998) *Social Science in Question*. London:Sage in association with the Open University.

Thomas J (2005) Issues for the future. In: Barrett G, Sellman D, Thomas J (eds) *Interprofessional Working in Health and Social Care: Professional Perspectives – An Introductory Text*. Basingstoke:Palgrave Macmillan,187–99.

Whittock M, Edwards C, McLaren S, Robinson O (2002) 'The tender trap': gender, part-time nursing and the effects of 'family-friendly' policies on career advancement. *Sociology of Health and Illness* 24(3):305–26.

WHO (1978) *Primary health care*. Report of the International Conference on Primary Health Care, Alma-Ata, USSR, 6–12 September 1978. *(Health for All Series No. 1)*. Geneva: World Health Organization.

Witz A (1992) *Professions and Patriarchy*. London:Routledge.

Organizational Issues

Tim Harle, Margaret Page and Yusuf Ahmad

Introduction

In this chapter, we focus on interprofessional working from an organizational perspective. In particular, we apply organizational theory to issues identified in the case-study material in Part I. We can view the current emphasis on interprofessional working in the context of new organizational forms and approaches to management and leadership that emphasize flat, rather than hierarchical, structures. In addition, workforce change in health and social care reflects wider changes in labour markets and patterns of work organization.

In a broad field, we bring two particular perspectives to bear. First, that of developments in the field of leadership within organizations. Secondly, that of complexity theory. Although the literature for the former is burgeoning, the latter is still growing: Haynes (2003) and Stacey and Griffin (2006) are examples which address the health sector.

In drawing on the case-study material, we indicate some parallels outside health care and promote a dialogue of learning from each other. As authors with differing backgrounds in business and the public sector, we have been prompted to engage in a debate around similarities and differences. A widely held view is offered by Flynn (2007:6): 'managing public services is not the same as managing services in the private sector'. While acknowledging significant areas of overlap, we cannot claim to have reached definitive agreement about such a statement. Our brief, which focuses on organizational issues, has not enabled us to explore in detail such questions as differing motivation.

However, we trust that the critical reflection and debate it has engendered has enriched our exploration.

Patient-centred approaches

An eclectic symposium on the future of the NHS (Tempest 2006) gathered 18 contributions from different professionals. After offering (sometimes conflicting) views from 17 practice areas, the final contribution asked, 'What do patients want?' At the start of our discussion, it is salutary to be reminded that, for all the concentration on links between different professions, we must not lose focus on the overarching purpose of our work. In Chapter 5, social worker(4) speaks of an 'extreme example … we failed her', with, literally, deadly consequences.

Service user(2) in Chapter 4 contrasts two experiences. A wasted initial pair of visits made her feel like an outsider as the different members of staff argued among themselves, while the second visit was 'absolutely brilliant'. The latter case involved bringing together the right professionals with the right information. We will explore the importance of information below.

The experiences of organizations that lose touch with what their customers want, exemplified in recent years by Marks & Spencer, are salutary. However, in the majority of cases in health and social care, the situation is exacerbated by the lack of alternative providers.

Disaggregation

The examples of patients being let down may be the consequence of separate parts of a system failing to work together. Consumers in recent years have become used to the idea of receiving services or goods without needing to worry about the internal organization or supply chains which deliver them. This trend has put pressure on those who traditionally act as brokers, whether of information or goods. Such disintermediation has been generally perceived as a good thing, although the experience of those who had booked flights directly with travel companies which failed during 2008 and were not covered by industry bonding schemes show that this is not a universal panacea.

ACTIVITY

Describe a situation in your experience where delivery of a service requires the patient to deal with constituent providers rather than a single service deliverer.

The experience of Service user(1) in Chapter 3 describes a situation more akin to managing individual elements than receiving a service. This is ironic, as

Service user(1) prefers holistic assessment. In the previous system, individual practitioners assessed her needs related only to their own area of work. Service user(1) described this as 'intrusive', as it entailed so many people visiting her home. Under the direct payment system, service users are allowed a great deal of leeway to organize their own services. However, the service user becomes the employer, with the accompanying obligations. To Service user(1), this is 'not all plain sailing. You have to take responsibility, you've got to hire and fire.'

If the consequences for the patient are more complicated, the same applies to the professionals. Community development worker in Chapter 3 describes how governance can become more convoluted:

> we're often working in big partnership groups often across the whole of [county] . . . [I] have sat on a whole series of review boards.

Not all this is beneficial, however: 'there's been an awful lot of consultation for the sake of it'. The whole question of differing accountabilities (blurred, contradictory, or subject to political whim) is one that is often raised in the context of differences between public- and private-sector management. Jessop (2003:1) suggests that there has been growing interest in the potential contribution of new forms of governance to solving co-ordination problems in and across a wide range of specialized social systems (such as the economy, and the legal, political and health systems) and civil society, and that this interest is reflected in growing ambiguities about the meaning of governance. He defines governance as the reflexive self-organization of independent actors involved in complex relations of reciprocal interdependence, with such self-organization being based on continuing dialogue and resource-sharing to develop mutually beneficial joint projects and to manage the contradictions and dilemmas inevitably involved in such situations. From this perspective, he argues that governance need not entail a complete symmetry in power relations or complete equality in the distribution of benefits: indeed, it is highly unlikely to do so, almost regardless of the object of governance or the 'stakeholders' who actually participate in the governance process. All that is involved in this preliminary definition is the commitment on the part of those involved to reflexive self-organization in the face of complex reciprocal interdependence.

Traditional and informal structures

'[M]ost of the work is done outside [the meeting].' Occupational therapist (OT)(1) in Chapter 1 highlights something that rings a bell with many. This is not the only example of the actual activity being different from the apparent. The same individual describes a big management attitude change, where 'the team are . . . almost moulding their manager'. Grint (2005:103–5) has observed something similar going on in the hierarchical world of the Royal

Air Force. He coined the term 'inverse learning' for the reversal of the traditional hierarchy between teacher and pupil.

ACTIVITY

In your work, do you observe lines of authority which do not coincide with formal structures? Are these acknowledged? What might account for the situations that do not
conform?

A good example of an inverted hierarchy is provided by Senior registrar, paediatrics (SRP) in Chapter 2:

> The better doctors, the more experienced doctors, *will do as they're told* – and so in that
> way it functions. Nurses know what they want and they often tell us what to do, and
> we do it. (emphasis added)

Emergency care consultant (ECC) in the same chapter has some interesting
observations on teams in an acute setting. Those who see themselves as the
top of a hierarchy feel that teamwork undermines their power or their self-
esteem: they fall back on their 'hierarchical cushion'. ECC rightly notes that
'Respect is something that is earned through a completely different process.'
We will be examining what promotes security and the conditions for emergence of such values as respect below.

Some of the issues highlighted have been found in many companies for
some time. Take the experience of OT(1) in Chapter 1:

> our management structure has changed . . . originally . . . we were managed by profes-
> sion, everybody had a professional hierarchical structure and we had a head of profes
> sion and then it went to the Chief Executive . . . so it was a very simple structure. Now
> . . . the district manager . . . he's my line manager, and then I have a clinical manager . . .
> who's an occupational therapist, so that's quite a big change.

The private sector is familiar with matrix organization, with tensions
between country and product managers, with organizing around customers.
But there remains a persistent view that there is an added degree of complexity
in areas such as health and social care, not least because of the political agenda.

An aspect that could be explored is that of differential power imbalances, in
terms not only of occupational and professional hierarchies, but also such considerations as gender and race. We discuss gender when considering organizational culture below, but saw no explicit references to race. It would be
interesting to explore how such power imbalances impact the efficacy of inter-

professional work. The literature on gender and race in terms of power imbalances is extensive, but tends to be perceived as a 'special interest' rather than integral to interprofessional and cross-boundary working. This perspective has been challenged by organizational researchers and consultants who assert that gender and race are reproduced in day-to-day organizational and leadership practices and reward systems, and theory (Acker 2006, Marshall 1995, Mills and Tancred 1992). This literature lends itself to a critique of linear approaches to change in favour of an understanding that is complex and emergent. From this perspective, improvization becomes a mindset for enacting leadership and change within complex networks of relationships (Fletcher 1998, Shaw 2002, Weick 1998).

One of many paradoxes is highlighted by Community development worker in Chapter 3:

> There's these things called compacts . . . something that the government has really enforced on all local authorities to produce. It's a voluntary agreement between statutory organizations and the voluntary sector.

The notion of a voluntary agreement being enforced illustrates the contradictions of today's environment.

Teamwork

The case studies in Part I illustrate the benefits of working in teams, but also the challenges that can occur for those who may be perceived as outsiders. The former is summed up by ECC in Chapter 2:

> teams make for safer patient care. When you have multiple people involved in a single process it gives you multiple checks.

A good example is described by social worker(3) in Chapter 5: being accompanied on a home visit was described as 'a bit of a luxury', yet this colleague was able to pick up on medication that was interacting. Summing up the situation, the social worker noted, 'if I'd gone out on my own I wouldn't necessarily have been aware of this'. Chapter 5 also offers an illustration of Belbin's (2004) team roles: 'chairman' is one of eight roles observed by Belbin in his schema for effective teams. Describing a meeting, Mental health nursing student(2) observed that

> the consultant was kind of chairing the meeting . . . she was struggling somewhat because she was controlling . . . I felt that maybe the ward manager should have chaired the meeting and given the consultant a chance to digest the information.

We can note how an outsider – in this case a student – may well be able to observe, if not always feel free to articulate, the obvious.

However, outsiders may have a sense of exclusion reinforced by strong teams. One of the researchers in Chapter 5 noted how nursing staff were sometimes reluctant to join ward-round meetings. This led the consultant to regard such behaviour as indicative of nurses' indifference to interprofessional practice – this was contradicted by their large attendance at a subsequent multidisciplinary workshop. We can hypothesize that what is described as 'safety in numbers' may have been at play. Sociologists and social anthropologists might speak in terms of tribal behaviour, and note how deviant behaviour is sometimes needed to break out across boundaries. This promotes development and learning, but is risky.

We will explore the importance of having points of security in times of uncertainty when considering leadership challenges around change below. At this stage, we can raise the question of what kind of leadership capacities need to be mobilised in interprofessional – and, increasingly, interorganizational and cross-sectoral contexts. Although our focus is on organizational rather than individual issues, we note how the articulations of various professionals quoted suggest an anxiety connected with issues of loss of identity, status or power. In particular, we believe that insights from psychology can help understand the leadership function. Attachment theory, associated especially with John Bowlby (1969), emphasizes the importance of a 'secure base' (originally observed between parent and child, but applicable to a wide range of relationships). It offers a framework for understanding the psychological impact of social and economic turbulence on communities and individuals. Kraemer and Roberts (1996) apply attachment theory to the social and political arena, acknowledging the widespread insecure attachment that is a feature of Western society. They argue that leaders need to address the attachment needs of individuals and communities, and the impact of insecurity and uncertainty that may be exacerbated by decision makers, themselves anxious to avoid anxiety caused by uncertainty. Within leadership studies, the notion of 'negative capability' as a quality of effective leadership in turbulent and uncertain times refers to the capacity to hold onto the anxiety of 'not knowing', while enabling and retaining the capacity to act thoughtfully and with responsibility (Simpson *et al.* 2002).

The role of place

A recurring theme in the case studies is how physical and spatial design can affect interprofessional working. The impact is exemplified by the contrasting experiences of Community nurse in Chapter 1:

> We've just moved offices and prior to the move . . . the professionals were separated from the support workers and it was quite difficult . . . the last two months since we have moved have been wildly different . . . It really is spot-on.

Other examples where close office location helped are offered by Health visitor in Chapter 3, who worked with a charity with a building adjacent to the clinic, and Senior midwife in Chapter 4, who commented how lucky she was to be in the middle of both key facilities and professionals.

Close office location by itself, however, does not guarantee better communication and teamworking. OT(1) in Chapter 1 notes the significance of an apparently trivial act:

> everybody leaves the door open and so we have quite a lot of conversation which is really helpful.

Nor do separate locations act as a barrier if the will is there:

> the physios are quite happy to come down and assess.
>
> (Adult nurse(2), Chapter 2)

Sarra (2006) offers a powerful narrative and reflection on the interplay between place and power in an NHS setting, informed by complexity theory. A corridor occupied by senior managers, known as 'the green mile', impacted a range of organizational issues from identity to performance management.

Boundaries

The very idea and language of interprofessional working implies boundaries, and yet this carries the danger that other boundaries – notably that with the patient – are relegated to secondary importance. Organizational theorists have much to learn from other disciplines. To take three examples:

- study of living systems demonstrates the importance of boundaries to promote healthy ecosystems, from cells to global populations,

- complexity theory illustrates how small changes in boundary conditions can lead to dramatic impacts,

- sociologists note the significance of liminal space in ritual and other activity.

In addition, leadership studies have shown a growing interest in such concepts as leading from the edge.

We can preface our investigation of the case-study material with a passage which sums up many of the key features we will examine.

> These complex networks of relationships offer very different possibilities for thinking about self and others. The very idea of boundaries changes profoundly. Rather than being a self-protective wall, boundaries become the place of meeting and exchange. We usually think of these edges as the means to define separateness, defining what's inside and what's outside. But in living systems, boundaries are something quite different. They are the place where new relationships take form, an important place of exchange and growth as an individual chooses to respond to another.
>
> (Wheatley 2005:48)

In an age where many advocate the importance of clarity – clear objectives, clear responsibilities – it is interesting to note the number of positive references to blurred barriers and overlap:

> we have a lot of blurred barriers . . . we do have quite clear overlaps.
>
> OT(1) Chapter 1

> If you look at the way that we work the roles are quite interchangeable so there are things where it is not clear whose responsibility it is.
>
> ECC, Chapter 2

> professional boundaries and differences are very much flattened and blurred, so although there are people here with years and years of experience and lots of qualifications and are much higher on the banding, for instance, than I am . . . we pretty much operate and treat each other as equal.
>
> Mental health nurse(1), Chapter 5

ACTIVITY

Can you identify roles which span boundaries in your area of practice? Are these formal or informal roles?

These experiences must be contrasted with others where boundaries appear to be firm. Health visitor in Chapter 1 quotes her experience:

> You'd never expect them [playworkers] to take responsibility for giving advice outside the remit that they are competent to do, because most of them work within specific competencies.

Where clinical or other expertise is called for, this is acceptable; however, a subsequent comment by the same health visitor suggests otherwise:

> I was never invited to any of their [GPs'] meetings – I didn't necessarily want to go, but they didn't seem to include geographically based people.

Note this example of a sense of exclusion identified above under a sociological perspective. Blurring of boundaries can also be perceived as a threat, as noted by GP in Chapter 1:

> Some doctors are a bit worried about this, I have heard doctors comment, 'Where is this going to end; are these nurses trying to be doctors?' We have to appreciate they are training up and there is a big overlap.

Social worker(2) in Chapter 2 feels there are difficulties around boundaries, describing how, in relation to a team, 'our roles are blurred because they will try to work around us'.

Lastly, we can note the pivotal role sometimes played organizationally by those who may be described as boundary spanners. In Chapter 2, Consultant geriatrician states how 'We all have our roles . . . [nurses] are a more direct bridge for the families.' This raises an important point about who is responsible to the patient, or consumer. This cannot be delegated to the customer relations department, but must be embedded within an organization. In this context, the experience of hard-pressed A&E staff as organizational representatives demonstrates parallels, albeit with differing degrees of acuteness, with staff at an airline check-in desk or in a bank's call centre.

Organizational culture

Classic texts, such as Schein (2004), describe the interplay between organizational culture and leadership, and offer tools and techniques for understanding the dynamics of organizations. Historically, an organization's culture has been seen as something that was driven 'top down', yet recent authors have offered a different perspective. Writing from the perspective of a business ethicist, Badaracco (1997) has noted the importance of everyday decisions and actions, where people get their hands dirty, while Harrison's (2007) autobiographical account of the agency staff industry is subtitled 'How Small Gestures Build Great Companies'. Neither uses the language of complexity theory, such as sensitivity to initial conditions and nonlinear dynamics (popularized as the 'butterfly effect'), and stability at far from equilibrium conditions (the so-called 'edge of chaos'). But both accounts are entirely in accord with its precepts, especially that of participative self-organization and emergence, where a whole system demonstrates features that are not observable in its constituent parts (the construction of temperature-controlled anthills is a favourite example from the natural world).

In business, a common cause for the failure of mergers and joint ventures to deliver the expected benefits is the difficulty of integrating organizational cultures. We see evidence of similar concerns in the case studies. In a multidisciplinary team setting, OT(1) in Chapter 1 describes '[what] people were very concerned about was that the council have a different style of management to the NHS'.

We also observed different cultures in different professions. For example, GP in Chapter 1 noted how

> nurses work much more from protocols than doctors and we know from out-of-hours' experience that nurses aren't disposed as much as doctors to be able to conclude something on the telephone.

In reflecting on such statements, it is instructive to consider the interplay between a number of factors, including professional standards, training regimes and individual expectations. Chapter 4 provides a vivid example of differing approaches between professions:

> The paediatricians are . . . very hot on doing lots of observations and things on babies . . . we did the minimum really with babies . . . leaving us to look at a baby and say, 'This is a well baby', 'This isn't a well baby'...I hate it. I think it's horrible.
>
> Community midwife(3)

Part I includes at least two significant examples of differing cultures, where different models may be at play:

- tensions between medical and social models around projects relating to disabled children in Chapter 3,

- differences between health and criminal justice systems relating to mental health care in Chapter 5.

Different expectations, desired outcomes, training, priorities, performance management systems, and regulatory regimes, among other factors, lead to differences of opinion among staff who see their roles in different ways. Our observations above surrounding interplay across boundaries are relevant here, expressed in memorable language by Mental health nurse(1) in Chapter 5: 'mongrels last longer than pedigree dogs'.

One contributor to culture is that of training. An observation from Manager in a large voluntary agency (MLVA) in Chapter 3 is pertinent:

> speech and language therapists [were sometimes asked] to approach things in a way that they had not been trained for . . . here they were asked just to respond to unexpected situations . . . This could be challenging; I don't think they were being defensive, but this was out of their territory.

The same individual draws attention to differences in organizational norms:

> Another factor was that some Trust members had quite boundaried roles; others had more autonomy; others were not able to make any decisions and had to take things back for further consultation.

Once again, an outsider is able to observe aspects of culture, which may be taken for granted by those enmeshed in them.

A particular aspect of organizational culture which is referred to on various occasions is that of attitudes to risk taking. Commenting on a difference between nurses and doctors referred to above, GP in Chapter 1 muses that 'it may be about risk taking'. Different attitudes to risk are also referred to by Psychologist in Chapter 5:

I think everybody would agree that risk isn't just to do with a mental disorder, you know, you have to look at a lot of other things as well.

==================== **ACTIVITY** ====================

Reflect on everyday incidents which have helped shape the culture of your workplace. How would you tell the story to others in different professional roles?

We can now turn to examples where organizational culture can be interpreted as the product of apparently insignificant events: an area that can be understood with insights from complexity theory, notably the concept of emergence. In the intermediate home-care setting described in Chapter 1, Community nurse described how

> [non-nursing professionals] might come across somebody who has been incontinent and would have to deal with it.

Such patient-centred learning experiences promote collaboration and teamwork. Chapter 4 provides an example of the law of unintended consequences, where midwives assisting in theatre

> came about because we don't have enough junior doctors to provide adequate cover in the middle of the night ... or to provide it within the confines of the European Working Time Directive ... we actually were doing fine until we had to reduce the length of hours that our juniors could be in hospital.
>
> Obstetric consultant(2)

Note, too, how this development occurred in a system that was perceived to be working well.

A debated question in considering organizational culture is the role that gender plays. There were relatively few explicit references to gender in the case studies. At least two of them appear to reflect rather simple stereotypes, albeit in a way which points to learning. In Chapter 2, ECC ventured:

> Dare I say it, I suspect that with increasing numbers of female doctors we will see increasingly better teamwork.

Meanwhile, in Chapter 4, we learn from obstetric consultant(2) that

> we occasionally get the odd problem with a newish junior doctor, often male [*laughs*] who insists on treating the midwives as nurses to do exactly as he tells them.

This consultant goes on to make a classic interprofessional point:

we say to our juniors, the midwives know far more than you guys [*sic*] know, and you must respect them and defer to them, they're *professionals in their own right*. (emphasis added)

One of the few explicit references to gender is made by MLVA in Chapter 3, who notes that

The interprofessional debates can also have a gender element as there are more men in youth work and more women working with younger children.

The use of information

Another common thread running through many of the case studies is the role played, for good or ill, by information. In particular, the sharing – or absence of sharing – of information is noted on various occasions. Some of these are mundane, but nevertheless useful, as illustrated by Community nurse in Chapter 1:

The documentation is all . . . one folder within the patient's home whilst they're under our care and one folder in our offices and we have a daily handover meeting.

However, the reverse is also true. As we saw when considering patient-centred approaches, failure to share information can have deadly consequences. Children's nurse in Chapter 2 is clearly frustrated:

And they [doctors] don't always write in the notes . . . Dreadful, dreadful communication . . . It's historical, it's ritual.

An anthropologist will note the use of tribal language.

The overworked adage that 'knowledge is power' finds some backing in the case studies. This may be viewed negatively, as by OT(1) in Chapter 1:

before, we had very clear information, and I think now under this different style of management we don't get all the information.

However, a positive view is expressed by Senior midwife in Chapter 4:

there's good communication between everybody . . . midwives certainly are given their full autonomy.

In this case, shared information promotes effective working. A good summary of the potential of information in patient care is provided by SRP in Chapter 3:

I think doctors give a lot of information. I was just talking to a consultant this morning, and she was talking, when I said, 'How do you interact with the service users?' She kept describing information she was giving.

In this context, it is important to note how even practical points such as the design of forms can have a deleterious effect, as noted in Chapter 1 by GP, who complains how the forms for sharing information on child protection and adults at risk from social services are not good for GPs.

From an organizational and leadership perspective, key questions to address include not simply the mechanics of information sharing (IT systems, forms), but awareness of the need to share information, and the willingness to do so among different professionals. Such attitudes are likely to be a reflection of organizational culture. In moving beyond a functional view of information, notions such as dialogue and reflexivity have the potential to improve inter-professional working (Isaacs 1993, Schein 1993). Critical reflection is often associated with self-awareness.

Leadership: alignment

We have sought to distil the implications for the leadership agenda into two themes. The first of these addresses many of the questions raised above under organizational culture. It also embraces performance management. If we were to choose one word to describe the key feature, it would be 'alignment'. A strong case can be made for choosing 'consistency' as an alternative; however, this runs the risk of being misinterpreted as ruling out creativity and innovation. This is paradoxical as, we argue, consistency promotes exactly the conditions where creativity and innovation thrive.

Chapter 1 provides a case in point. Referring to some social workers, Health visitor says

> I don't think they mean to be obstructive. They just . . . their priorities aren't necessarily the same as ours.

The same person refers to a typical example of a performance management system where it is a moot point whether it is encouraging the most appropriate behaviour:

> Relatively recently . . . [GPs] realized that if we did the immunizations then they would get extra money.

The track record of the NHS – from 48-hour GP appointment targets to new dentists' contracts – provides further examples of the law of unintended consequences. Although it is beyond the scope of this chapter, examining motivation might provide salutary lessons. From a leadership perspective, the promotion of aligned targets – and the dissemination of information about them – are vital.

Such considerations are particularly apposite in the voluntary sector, where coercion (in its neutral sense) is less likely. Indeed, Chapter 3 provides examples. First, Community development worker highlights different time horizons:

The worst thing about it is probably this short-termism.

Then, MLVA detects inconsistencies:

> There was considerable 'in principle' support from the local social services managers but this was not necessarily seen as a priority at more senior levels.

This last manager also highlights an instance where national training guidelines appeared to be inconsistent with the approach being encouraged:

> They also seemed to have very different polces and expectations in relation to inter-agency collaboration...looking at some health visitor training guidelines from the Department of Health, I was really surprised that it said the HV [health visitor] role is to be THE lead professional around early years and to make things happen in their locality, to instruct [sic] other people . . . there was no mention of partnership or collaboration . . . It gave the strong view that they were the only leaders.

Lastly, we can note a scenario when measuring the wrong thing promotes sub-optimal (at best) behaviour. In Chapter 1, GP describes an experience familiar to many:

> Huge problems and around the waiting list problem. We spend a lot of time trying to be the patients' advocate. There was a lot of messing around with certain types of patient. Failed paperwork, people being sent out too early and bouncing back in too readily.

Here is an illustration of the need for an integrated approach; in particular, the performance management regime (including measurement) should capture the whole system – the patient experience – and align behaviours and organizational culture. Too often, systems measure what is easy to measure.

ACTIVITY

Contrast examples of aligned and non-aligned performance management systems you have experienced. Highlight common themes in examples of good and bad practice.

In addition to such explicit considerations as performance management systems, we can also refer back to the importance of small things in promoting organizational culture. The contrast between traditional and emergent approaches is provided by the most successful airline in the USA in the past generation. On leaving Southwest Airlines to join rival start-up JetBlue, the Executive Vice-President of Human Resources noted how 'Values were central at Southwest Airlines, but they just happened. I think it's better to decide upfront what they'll be' (quoted in Gittell 2005:226). Just happened? We doubt it. Reports of Southwest's early years emphasize the overwhelming consistency – by no means in a traditional vein – from founder Herb Kelleher and colleagues.

To borrow a phrase from complexity theory, this consistency in leadership could be described as fractal – consisting of repeating patterns that are seen distributed at different levels in an organization.

Leadership: change

Our final group of observations revolve around a pervasive agenda: that of change. This positioning is deliberate. In contrast to traditional approaches to change management – a term which is one of the great oxymorons of our age – we believe that the focus should be on creating the conditions for change. Once more, we can learn from nature and the work of two pioneering biologists: 'Maturana and Varela note something quite important for our activities with one another. We can never direct a living system. We can only disturb it' (Wheatley and Kellner-Rogers 1999:49). In contrast to traditional Newtonian perspectives of cause and effect, insights from complexity theory encourage participative self-organization and emergence (Harle 2007).

This approach involves revisiting notions of control from a leadership perspective. ECC in Chapter 2 furnishes some interesting observations. The scene of an accident may be 'quite complicated and quite uncontrolled', yet 'the actual lines of who is in charge are quite clear'. Acute circumstances accelerate team development: 'you are with people you have never met before and have to form teams in a very short space of time'. Hardly a surprising observation, but it is interesting to note the consultant's observation that 'the determination to keep control can be undermining to the quality of care'. This appears to be an exemplar of a contemporary trend in military strategy noted by Grint (2005:38). Mission Command has its origins in mid-nineteenth-century Prussia: a system of leadership made up of 'general directives, not specific orders, strategic aims not operational requirements, thereby enabling decentralized control that facilitated distributed leadership and the ability of local ground commanders to seize the initiative rather than await orders'. Streatfield (2001) examines the paradox of control from a complexity theory perspective, based on his experience in the pharmaceutical sector.

The importance of a secure base in times of uncertainty is well illustrated by Health visitor in Chapter 1:

> There's been a lot of change and a lot of insecurity, so health visitors are . . . desperately trying to hold on to what they know they can do, and not wanting others to do assessments for them, etcetera, keeping that responsibility. And that's quite difficult when you've got a multiprofessional team, and you're meant to be working together.

Although beyond the scope of this chapter, we can consider suggestive parallels with the work of psychologists such as Ainsworth and Bowlby, referred to above, on attachment and promoting a secure base. Two contrasting quotes describe feelings of security and anxiety encountered in the case studies:

> I feel comfortable in my role and secure in what I am doing so it doesn't matter.
>
> ECC, Chapter 2

> It's quite difficult for health visitors to know what their actual role is . . . health visitors have generally felt really quite insecure about where they're meant to be going.
>
> Health visitor, Chapter 3

ACTIVITY

Note down occasions where you have felt confident to ask questions in a work group. If you felt inhibited from asking questions, what contributed to this?

Edmondson *et al.* (2001) provide observations from the field of cardiac surgery, where 'zones of psychological safety' promote team learning. They mention in particular the need for open questioning: their work is paralleled in the experience of ECC in an acute care setting in Chapter 2:

> we rely on the nursing staff to work with the medical staff to flag up issues and problems so one of the key features – it is a bit like the crew resource management issues in aviation – is to *create a safe environment*. So we empower the staff – 'Are you sure about that? Is that the right thing to do?' – to ask questions. And therefore the student nurse can ask the consultant, in an open atmosphere – ' . . . Why are you doing that?' (emphasis added)

In considering the case-study material, we have noted a number of paradoxes. In closing this review of leadership in the context of interprofessional health care, we can note the research of Collins (2001:20), whose prosaic description of a 'Level 5 executive' describes one who 'builds enduring greatness through a paradoxical blend of personal humility and professional will'.

Summary

Our exploration of the case-study material in Part I has identified a number of recurring themes.

First, we have noted a number of paradoxes. Some can have positive outcomes, as where blurred responsibilities can improve patient care, despite the call for more precise accountabilities. But we have also identified aspects of paradox and contradiction in both the espoused rhetoric of interprofessional work and the practice of it. In a situation where professional hierarchies continue to be reinforced in terms of reward and power, the aspirations towards flatter, more participative structures remain just that.

Secondly, we have noted differing perspectives on the degree of similarity and difference between public- and private-sector leadership. We trust that our own critical debates and comments around leadership will provide a fruitful source for reflection, learning and development.

Mention of the public and private sectors leads to a third theme: that of boundaries. Here we can point to the positive aspect of interaction and developments across boundaries. But we must also raise the irony that focus in the inter-professional agenda on work between professions might draw attention away from the most significant boundary of all – that between patient and carers.

Which brings us to a final theme: that whatever perspectives can be brought to bear, the challenge for all professionals is to ensure that the organization works for the patient.

References

Acker J (2006) Inequality regimes: gender, class and race in organizations. *Gender and Society* 20(4):441–6.

Badaracco J (1997) *Defining Moments.* Boston:Harvard Business School Press.

Belbin R (2004) *Management Teams: Why They Succeed or Fail.* (2nd edn) Oxford:Elsevier.

Bowlby J (1969) *Attachment and Loss: Vol 1. Attachment.* New York:Penguin.

Collins J (2001) *Good to Great.* London:Random House.

Edmondson A, Bohmer R, Pisano G (2001) Speeding up team learning. *Harvard Business Review* 79(9):125–32.

Fletcher J (1998) Relational practice: a feminist reconstruction of work. *Journal of Management Inquiry* 7(2):163–86.

Flynn N (2007) *Public Sector Management.* (5th edition) London:Sage.

Gittell J (2005) *The Southwest Airlines Way.* New York:McGraw-Hill.

Grint K (2005) *Leadership: Limits and Possibilities.* Basingstoke:Palgrave Macmillan.

Harle T (2007) The prairie and the rainforest: ecologies for sustaining organizational change. *Business Leadership Review* 4(3):1–15.

Harrison S (2007) *The Manager's Book of Decencies.* New York:McGraw-Hill.

Haynes P (2003) *Managing Complexity in the Public Services.* Maidenhead:Open University Press.

Isaacs W (1993) Taking flight: dialogue, collective thinking, and organizational learning. *Organizational Dynamics* 22(2):24–39.

Jessop B (2003) *Governance and Metagovernance: On Reflexivity, Requisite Variety, and Requisite Irony.* Lancaster University. www.lancs.ac.uk/fass/sociology/papers/jessop-governance-and-metagovernance.pdf

Kraemer S, Roberts J (eds) (1996) *The Politics of Attachment.* London:Free Association Books.

Marshall J (1995) *Women Managers Moving On.* London:Routledge.

Mills A, Tancred P (1992) *Gendering Organisational Analysis.* London:Sage.

Sarra N (2006) The emotional experience of performance management in the health sector: the corridor. In: Stacey R, Griffin D (eds) *Complexity and the Experience of Managing Public Sector Organizations.* Abingdon:Routledge,81–107.

Schein E (1993) On dialogue, culture, and organizational learning. *Organizational Dynamics* 22(2):40–51.

Schein E (2004) *Organizational Culture and Leadership.* (3rd edition) San Francisco:Jossey-Bass.

Shaw P (2002) *Changing Conversations in Organizations.* Abingdon:Routledge.

Simpson P, Harvey C, French R (2002) Leadership and negative capability. *Human Relations* 55(10):1209–26.

Stacey R, Griffin D (eds) (2006) *Complexity and the Experience of Managing Public Sector Organizations.* Abingdon:Routledge.

Streatfield P (2001) *The Paradox of Control in Organizations.* Abingdon:Routledge.

Tempest M (ed.) (2006) *The Future of the NHS.* St Albans:XPL.

Weick K (1998) Improvisation as a mindset for organizational analysis. *Organization Science* 9(5):543–55.

Wheatley M (2005) *Finding Our Way.* San Francisco:Berrett-Koehler.

Wheatley M, Kellner-Rogers M (1999) *A Simpler Way* San Francisco:Berrett-Koehler.

11

Values and Ethics in Interprofessional Working

Derek Sellman

Introduction

When, after two years of disappointing performances and results, the England football team put on an impressive display to beat Croatia in Zagreb in September 2008, many commentators expressed the opinion that the turn-around in fortunes occurred because individual players put aside their personal aspirations in order to focus on their contribution to the team. Perhaps some-what counter-intuitively, this resulted in some players putting in their best individual international performance of recent times. In the aftermath of the match, it was the coach who was credited with making a positive difference by generating an ethic in which individuals played for each other and for the benefit of the team, rather than merely for themselves. Similar features emerge in the accounts of effective and ineffective interprofessional working from social and health care professionals presented earlier in this book. As the obstetric consultant (2) (female) in Chapter 4 states:

> It's kind of crazy not to use . . . expertise . . . anybody who can contribute anything, it's all gratefully received and that's fine.

In Chapter 3 the manager of a large voluntary agency (MLVA) reflects on dif-ferences in interprofessional working in two similar units:

> there was quite a difference in their approach and level of engagement although they were working for the same health trust with the same managers. *Some things are about*

individuals, some things about informal leadership and the way people were supervised and their accountability structures, these vary a lot between different professionals. (emphasis added)

Illustrations such as these point to a number of conditions which I believe are needed if interprofessional working is to be effective. In this chapter I will begin to explore three of these conditions, which emerged from my analysis of material in Part I:

1 The Willingness Condition: the willingness to do whatever is required to contribute to effective teamworking. This includes a willingness to put the needs of the team on an equal, if not higher, footing than personal needs.
2 The Trust Condition: the recognition that effective teamworking requires professionals to trust one another.
3 The Leadership Condition: the recognition that effective teamworking requires effective leadership.

By definition interprofessional collaboration requires teamworking, and this is as true for those working in social and health care as it is for those working in any other field of collaborative endeavour. Indeed there would seem to be more that unites than divides the values and ethics guiding social and health care practice. Those in receipt of social and health care (as well as those who have not yet been socialized into particular professional perspectives) can be reasonably supposed to expect social care and health care workers to subscribe to a common set of values and ethics. This expectation is reflected in the code of practice governing social care professionals in the UK, drawn up by the General Social Care Council (GSCC 2002); and in the codes of conduct governing UK health care professionals, developed by the General Medical Council (GMC 2006) for medicine, the Nursing and Midwifery Council (NMC 2008) for nursing and midwifery, and the Health Professions Council (HPC 2008) for 13 other health professions. In any case, the goals of social and health professions relate to the pursuit of human betterment, what Sockett calls the 'ideal of service' (1993:16); although this idea has been discredited; both in sociology, where such altruistic sentiments are often dismissed as serving professional self-interests, and (perhaps more insidiously) through government imperatives concerned primarily with targets, albeit with a recent nod to ideas of customer care.

Despite such attacks, professional aspirations as expressed in the various professional codes continue to subscribe to some form of ideal of service, and this alone should provide a foundation from which all social and health care professional groups might agree about the operation of their claimed values and ethics. Yet, those who work in the social and health care services will recognize that while there exists agreement in general between different professional groups about the overall purpose(s) of work for human betterment, professions may interpret differently the operational specifics of any given value or ethical tenet, what Pecukonis *et al.* (2008) describe as profession-centrism.

Approaches to ethics

One way to categorize ethics is to make a distinction between act-based and agent-based ethics. Act-based ethics takes the position that what is important is the action taken in any given situation, and this focus can be found in the moral theories of consequentialism and deontology, as well as in the princi-plism derived from these types of theories. Briefly, consequentialist theories start from the premise that what is good is determined by how far the conse-quences contribute to the greater good, and derive primarily from the work of John Stuart Mill (1806–73); the concern with consequences (ends) rather than actions (the means by which outcomes are achieved) is one defining feature of consequentialist theories. In contrast, deontological, or duty-based, theories assume that the goodness of an action is determined by how far the act conforms with fulfilling duty, and the measure of morality lies in the means (the actions) rather than in the ends (the outcomes of actions). Deontology is famously associated with Immanuel Kant (1724–1804).

Principlism is an approach to ethics championed by Beauchamp and Childress (2001) that focuses on general principles supported from more than one moral theory. These principles are derived primarily from consequentialist and deontological theories, giving rise to the suspicion that those two theories are more closely aligned than is usually acknowledged. Thus 'respect for autonomy' finds support, albeit for different reasons, from the theoretical per-spectives of both Kant and Mill. In this way, according to proponents, princi-plism offers a practical guide to moral action and helps to overcome the purported impasse when deontology clashes with consequentialism. For this reason principlism has become popular as an action-guiding approach to ethical practice among health (if not social) care professionals.

The four principles of Beauchamp and Childress are: respect for autonomy; beneficence (to do good); non-maleficence (to do no harm); and (distribu-tive) justice.

Act-based ethics also finds support from the values that underpin human rights, and it is social care professionals (more than health care professionals) whose code of practice is most explicitly focused on issues of human rights (GSCC 2002). Nevertheless, human rights are not entirely inconsistent with agent-centred approaches to ethics, and it is to these I now turn.

In contrast to act-based approaches, agent-based ethics focuses on the person rather than (or as well as) the action. So in agent-centred ethics, the character of the person is as important as the action. Agent-centred ethics implies that individuals have, or have developed, particular characteristics (or virtues) from which actions are derived. Thus virtue ethics is agent-centred and generally assumes that individuals will act characteristically in ways consis-tent with their virtues. Far from failing to offer a guide to action (as critics of virtue ethics suggest), virtues are action-guiding. As Hursthouse (1997) reminds us, the person who has the virtue of courage will act in courageous ways, just as the honest person acts honestly. Following Aristotle (1953 edn) and MacIntyre (1985) I have argued that honesty, justice, courage, trustworthiness and open-mindedness are primary virtues for the practice of nursing (Sellman 2000, 2003, 2006, 2007) and by extension, for other social care and health care practices. Professional practitioners acting characteristically from the value base these virtues imply are motivated not only to act in ways that promote the flourishing of individual clients and patients, but also to recognize the need (and act so as) to develop the necessary competencies required for their specific professional practice. Virtue ethics does not claim the status of a moral theory as such – it is more of a general approach to living (and practising) well – so the question is not so much how should an individual practitioner act in any particular situation, rather it is what sort of person should the practitioner strive to become.

ACTIVITY

Can you think of a time when you were surprised by the actions of someone you know well? Write brief notes on what happened and what it was exactly that surprised you; also try to work out why you found it so surprising.

One significant feature of the distinction between act- and agent-based ethics, particularly for practitioners, is that the person aiming for virtue in the right measure will, generally speaking, act in concert with their inclinations, while the individual attempting to act in concert with the requirements either of that which leads to the best outcome (consequentialism) or of duty (deontology) may find many of their actions contrary to their inclinations. If you attempted the last Activity you may have found that the origin of your surprise was that the person acted uncharacteristically. If so, it lends credence to the idea that, on the whole, people have some fairly fixed ways of behaving and, further, that they tend to act in ways consistent with their characters.

The Willingness Condition

The Willingness Condition is the willingness to do whatever is required to contribute to effective teamworking. This includes a willingness to put the needs of the team on an equal, if not higher, footing than personal needs in order that the team can best meet the needs of clients:

> If you mention social workers to health visitors they all go, 'Oh, God, they never respond' . . . I don't think they mean to be obstructive . . . their priorities aren't necessarily the same as ours.
>
> Health visitor, Chapter 1

According to Couturier *et al.* (2008:342), 'social workers, psychologists, nurses and doctors, for example, are epistemologically distinct professional groups [which is] . . . an unavoidable condition of their work'. In other words, to be a social worker, a nurse, a doctor, or other health and social care practitioner is to have the appropriate knowledge and skill set for that particular professional role. Moreover, that skill set comes with, and emerges from, a particular professional culture with its own set of antecedents. As discussed in Chapter 6, pursuing the idea that each professional group has its own cultural heritage that can hinder interprofessional working, Pecukonis *et al.* (2008:424) suggest that 'Perhaps the first and most important step in developing interprofessional cultural competence is a *willingness* to enter into a dialogue with another professional' (emphasis added). By interprofessional cultural competence they mean demonstrating respect for the cultural traditions of other professional groups and being open to valuing the contribution(s) those other groups can make to the care of service users. A willingness to engage with other individual practitioners from other professional groups can be stifled by the uncritical acceptance of stereotypes such as the one intimated by the comments of the health visitor above.

=============================== **ACTIVITY** ===============================

Try to identify someone who seems (to you at least) to act as if they know it all. Sketch out one or two examples that illustrate the point that they really do not know it all.

The need to engage with other health and social care professionals (and others involved in care delivery) is illustrated by the point forcefully made by Irvine *et al.* (2002) who note that it is difficult to imagine that a single profession (or a single individual professional) can ever know or do everything to meet all the social and/or health care needs of any one client or patient. Accordingly there is, they claim, a moral obligation to work collaboratively with other caregivers in pursuit of serving the best interests of clients.

The first part of the willingness condition is a willingness to accept the need to maintain, update and develop one's skills. This requires a degree of humility in acknowledging that there are things one does not yet know or that one cannot yet do; what Race (2006) calls the 'transit box' in his competency model. The transit box is useful, for in it will be the things that a practitioner knows that they cannot yet do and that they do not yet know; and armed with this knowledge the practitioner can instigate an action plan to overcome the identified knowledge and skill shortfalls. However, in Race's model there is a further 'danger box' inhabited by those things one does not know one does not know (or cannot do); this is a danger, for obvious reasons. If a practitioner is unaware of a shortfall in their skills then they may put clients at risk by acting on the basis of incomplete knowledge. This undermines the values of beneficence and non-maleficence. The driver who does not know the rules of negotiating a roundabout and yet believes he is a good driver is clearly a danger to other road users; and the danger comes directly from his lack of insight. If you tried the Activity above then you may have identified a practitioner who thinks of themselves as a good practitioner but who fails to recognize their own shortfalls. Of course, these shortfalls are invisible to the self and the only way to find out about them is to ask others; this requires a further willingness to actively listen to and act upon what those others tell you about your knowledge and skill set.

Unfortunately, individuals who think they know it all tend not to ask others about their own performance precisely because they lack insight into their own failings. This poses a serious problem for interprofessional working. On this account a competent practitioner needs to have, maintain and develop the necessary skills for their particular professional practice. In order to convert effective uniprofessional practice into effective interprofessional practice it is necessary to acknowledge that it is not simply a matter of being good at and getting on with one's job. It requires a willingness to acknowledge the need to adapt one's skills so that they make the most effective contribution to the team. Just as the poor team performances of the England football players before their victory in Croatia did not reflect their individual skills, so too it is possible that the combined efforts of even the most skilled social and health care practitioners may not result in effective interprofessional collaboration. The comment of the Health visitor in Chapter 1 about the collective view health visitors hold of social workers quoted at the beginning of this section illustrates the point. Each professional may demonstrate their uniprofessional skills, but without a willingness to work out how best to make their respective skills work for the team, the overall performance (the effects on service users) will leave something to be desired.

In other words, there is a need for individual practitioners to be willing to subordinate their personal and/or professional aspirations to the goals of the team. Thus the willingness to co-operate, collaborate and compromise becomes self-evident. The comments of the Occupational therapist (OT)(1) in Chapter 1 support this when she says:

> the *teamworking* is more important than their professional role or . . . status . . . We'll link with anybody if it's in the best interests of the client.

This is further reflected in the comments of the community nurse in the same chapter:

> If there's a therapy programme that needs doing . . . rather than sending in two or three different people then the nurse will actually follow the therapy programme as well.

These two practitioners appear comfortable with other professionals getting involved in what otherwise would be considered uniprofessional tasks.

In addition to a willingness to subordinate personal or professional aspirations to the goals of the team, effective interprofessional working also requires a willingness to acknowledge the contribution of other professionals, a willingness to recognize one's own limitations, and a willingness to engage in genuine dialogue with other points of view. This is the kind of thing Pecukonis *et al.* (2008) have in mind as part of interprofessional cultural competence. The lack of willingness to engage with other professionals is how the Health visitor in Chapter 1 perceives 'never [being] invited to any of their [GP] meetings'. The key to this kind of willingness lies in the development of what I have described elsewhere as the virtue of open-mindedness (Sellman 2003). To be open-minded in this sense is to be open to the possibility that one may be wrong not only about one's firmly held beliefs but also to the possibility that one's actions may be based on faulty reasoning or evidence. This willingness is reflected by the emergency care consultant (ECC) in Chapter 2 who claims to be open to questions about his decisions:

> So we empower the staff . . . to ask questions. And therefore the student nurse can ask the consultant, in an open atmosphere – ' . . . Why are you doing that?'

This suggests the consultant is comfortable with uncertainty and comfortable with explaining and justifying his decisions. This consultant clearly has democratic tendencies and is comfortable with some blurring of the boundaries between different professional groups.

However, the personal willingness of professionals to engage with one another can be obstructed by structural, procedural and cultural barriers. Hence, while the personal characteristics of practitioners are important in meeting the willingness condition, the blame for failures in interprofessional working cannot be laid solely on the shoulders of individual professionals. For Couturier *et al.* (2008), the epistemologies of different professional groups get in the way of effective collaboration; and for Kvarnstrom (2008:19), 'difficulties [are] related to the influence of the surrounding organization'. While Kvarnstrom is suggesting the problem lies with whether or not professionals feel they get the appropriate support from the organization, there is a more trenchant problem when the organizational culture discourages rather than encourages the kind of innovation that effective interprofessional working requires. This can happen unintentionally and is reflected in the words of the psychiatrist in Chapter 5:

> There is a split in my view between the nursing staff and everybody else, and it has been extremely difficult to get the nursing staff to share the vision in the same way as the rest of the multidisciplinary team.

This individual seems to be implying that the nurses are unwilling at a professional or personal level, whereas an alternative view, and one that reflects a structural problem, is voiced by OT(2) in the same chapter, who recognizes this apparent unwillingness of the nurses to be an understandable response to a blame culture:

> And, because of the blame culture, the discipline *(nursing)* is increasingly retreating into themselves. You know, the nurses start being particularly blamed and . . . it's extremely difficult for them to sort of maintain their prominence and significance in the multidisciplinary team . . . There is a fear of actually engaging in the multidisciplinary process because that is a potential for further blame.

In MacIntyre's (1985) analysis this would be a symptom of institutional dominance, while Potter (2002) would understand this as failure of the organization to recognize that ethical practice can only thrive in an ethical organization.

The Trust Condition

The Trust Condition is the recognition that effective teamworking requires professionals to trust one another.

> You have to trust people to be doing the right thing.
> ECC, Chapter 2

According to Pullon (2008), trust between professionals (along with uniprofessional competence and respect) is a prerequisite for effective interprofessional working. And while the willingness of individual professionals to trust one another is a personal attribute of practitioners that we are right to encourage, trust can only flourish in a climate of trust (Sellman 2006), and a climate of trust relies on more than the willingness of individual practitioners to trust one another. As Potter (2002) notes, trust requires institutional arrangements to be trustworthy and to encourage rather than discourage trust among individuals.

─────────────── **ACTIVITY** ───────────────

Presumably there are social and health care professionals you would trust and those you would not. Make a list of those you trust and those you distrust in a social or health care setting and try to write something about what it is that makes a professional trustworthy or untrustworthy. Reflect on the basis for your opinion of the relative trustworthiness of different professionals. Is it based on personal experience, media portrayal, defence of your own profession, or something else entirely?

I have rehearsed elsewhere the important role trust and trustworthiness play in professional practice (Sellman 2006, 2007), and this is reflected in the stories related by the practitioners in earlier chapters in this book. The ECC quoted above goes on to indicate that some of his colleagues have been reluctant to allow other professionals to undertake tasks traditionally reserved for doctors; one reason for this may be that the doctors do not think other professionals can be trusted to do the task effectively. Of course, trust is earned rather than given, and for practitioners to trust one another it is necessary for each to show that not only can they perform their uniprofessional role effectively but also that they can be trusted, as and when appropriate, with tasks traditionally the preserve of a different profession. This kind of trust is evident in the comments of the occupational therapist (OT1) in Chapter 1:

> I deal with physiotherapy quite a lot . . . and (the physio) does a lot of postural management and seating.

Clearly, in this scenario each trusts the other not only to take on what might otherwise be uniprofessional specific tasks, but also to know when to call upon the specialist expertise of the other. In other words, where there is a blurring of boundaries, any professional who takes on any task must be able to demonstrate a satisfactory level of skill for that task. This does pose a dilemma for professional identity, but if interprofessional working involves the blurring of task boundaries then not only must professionals be willing to accept they may need to take on roles for which their primary professional role did not prepare them (which requires a willingness to develop new competencies), but also they must be willing to accept that some of their cherished professional roles or tasks may be undertaken by those with different disciplinary training and qualifications. As such, interprofessional working requires individual professionals to satisfy the willingness condition.

Demonstrating the appropriate level of skill and satisfying the willingness condition in this way may help to explain the development of trust between individual practitioners from different professionals, and may reflect a fairly standard pattern of relationship development of group members in the transition into teams. But it may remain at the personal level and be the exception rather than the rule. As O'Neill (2002) reminds us, we do not concern ourselves with the inherent contradiction of distrusting in the abstract while trusting in the particular. To use one of her examples, we may distrust estate agents in general, but when we want to sell our house we will do our best to find an estate agent we can trust, and we may go about this by seeking personal recommendations. It is not unreasonable to assume something similar is going on in relation to trust between different professional groups: the way the social worker in Chapter 1 describes a lack of trust of nurses may occur in both directions, yet there may be specific situations in which a particular nurse and a particular social worker will learn to trust one another.

Failures of uniprofessional skill or of the willingness condition will quickly erode trust between practitioners and very likely lead to frustration and irritation. This is illustrated by social worker(1) in Chapter 1 who, in complaining about the nurses' failure to ensure that the transport services were aware of the patient's condition, expresses her frustration at the futility of all of her earlier efforts to get the patient home with all the necessary services in place by saying, 'Sometimes you feel as although you have to treat everyone as although they're stupid.' This frustration of one professional about another's role performance is unlikely to induce future trust between the two; and it is possible that distrust of one member of a particular profession may become generalized into stereotypical labelling of a whole profession as a group not to be relied on, or to be the cause of much of the problems when interprofessional working goes badly.

I have noted elsewhere that 'Just as trust flourishes in a climate of trust, so distrust flourishes in a climate of distrust' (Sellman 2006:113), and as the lack of trust between professional groups (or between individual professionals from different professional groups) increases, so it becomes harder to generate a climate of trust in which professionals might (re)learn to trust one another. If, having once lost trust, professionals have any chance of regaining trust between professionals, then each must meet the willingness condition; that is, each professional must be open to the possibility that they may be wrong to distrust a practitioner of a different professional group (or indeed a whole professional group in general). And this is another example of the need to satisfy the willingness condition.

Where trust relationships break down, as seems to be the case with the social worker quoted above, it is possible that trust can be restored, but it is likely to emerge initially at the individual level and it might then proceed in ever-widening circles of generalization, at least to the point at which distrust proves to be warranted.

Imagine that the social worker in the scenario described above takes a new position in a different part of the country, having arrived in the new practice area with a stereotypical view of nurses as practitioners who are not to be trusted. She is surprised to find one nurse who, against expectation, turns out to be rather good at his job (that is, demonstrates his uniprofessional skill), and consequently warrants both respect as a professional in his own right and trust as a fellow professional with a valuable contribution to make to service delivery. As our social worker spends more time in this area she finds there are other nurses just as competent and professional as this first nurse, and finally realizes that all the registered nurses here can be trusted to work as part of a team with a focus on the needs of the patients. Our social worker has now moved from a general distrust of nurses to a specific position about the trustworthiness of the nurses in a particular practice area.

In effect she has moved from holding the view that '*in general nurses are not to be trusted*' to '*in general, nurses are not to be trusted, but nurses working in this particular practice area can be trusted*'. As long as our social worker continues to encounter nurses who demonstrate their expected uniprofessional skill set, then it is not difficult to imagine that she will generalize further to the view that '*in general nurses can be trusted*'. This might take a long time, but if this progression of trust continues then the original formulation that '*nurses cannot be trusted*' will become redundant and in need of revision to reflect the changed opinion the social worker now has of the trustworthiness of nurses in general. However, it may not be necessary for that level of generalization to be reached for effective interprofessional working in any given department or situation.

Of course, social workers may not be trusted in relation to specific issues by other health and social care professionals. The general practitioner in Chapter 1 says:

> doctors are worried about confidentiality; there are huge issues about, 'What can I tell the social worker, I know there is a risk here . . . but what ball will it start rolling?' These were the sort of issues that people would bring to coffee-time discussions. What can I tell social services; what action would I be entering into? There is no room for an off-the-record discussion.

It appears that doctors may be reluctant to share information with social workers because they (social workers) are obligated to proceed in predetermined ways when they become party to certain sorts of information. If one feature of interprofessional collaboration is the sharing of information, then this kind of distrust between professionals becomes a barrier to effective interprofessional working. Sharing information appropriately has been recognized as particularly problematic in interprofessional and inter-agency working, and guidelines for practitioners and managers have therefore been produced (HM Government 2008).

There are, however, complexities which need to be addressed in this regard. As mentioned earlier, there are codes governing the way that all health and social care professionals behave in the UK. However, a profession may, in addition, have particular professional obligations which may not always align with those of another profession. For example, midwives must also abide by rules specifically governing midwifery practice (NMC 2004), which state that midwives must respect and support women's wishes for care (for example, having a baby at home), even if these wishes do not accord with medical or midwifery recommendations. On the other hand, doctors are obliged to 'protect patients from risk of harm posed by another colleague's conduct, performance or health. The safety of patients must come first at all times' (GMC 2006:23). There have been a number of occasions when individual midwives have found themselves facing disciplinary procedures because they have supported women's wishes and have subsequently been deemed by colleagues or employers to have compromised patient safety (Laurance 1999, AIMS 2004).

In these sorts of situations, it is not surprising that practitioners may hesitate about sharing information with their colleagues from other disciplines. Moreover, all health and social care professionals are bound to respect client confidentiality, except in cases where individuals are at risk of serious harm, or serious criminal activity is involved (HM Government 2008). A key issue affecting confidentiality, however, is that its maintenance depends on individual practitioners' subjective judgements about whether or not risks or criminal activities are 'serious'. Therefore, where a professional perceives that information will be used by another practitioner to a client's (or their own) disadvantage, owing to conflicting professional perspectives or loyalties, there is often little likelihood that effective interprofessional working involving exchange of information will occur.

Building trust between members of the interprofessional team is therefore crucial, if they are going to work together constructively. A key factor is that practitioners understand differences between their own and colleagues' priorities, perspectives and professional obligations. The MLVA in Chapter 3 describes the strategy that her organization employs in this regard:

> *'How did confidentially issues get resolved?'*
> Different tactics really, clear guidelines on how to make referrals . . . we identified link people like duty team managers who would understand where the agency was coming from. Also training, going to social work team meetings, mutual information sharing . . . we had a system where at inter-agency team meetings people took it in turns to talk about their roles and it was open to anyone working or funded by Sure Start to participate. Different professions would take the agenda for half an hour and share what they thought others needed to know about their service and interprofessional or inter-agency dilemmas and issues.

The Leadership Condition

The Leadership Condition is the recognition that effective teamworking requires effective leadership. Leadership is important and is discussed in other parts of this book (see, in particular Chapters 8, 9 and 10). Here I will just offer a few brief comments.

=== **ACTIVITY** ===

Think of someone you have come across who you consider either an excellent or an ineffective leader. Make some notes about what it is that makes that person, in your opinion, either excellent or ineffective at leading others.

That a team needs a leader seems self-evident and, consistent with the willingness condition discussed above, there is a requirement to accept that the leadership role at any particular time will be best undertaken by the most suitable person for that occasion. In other words, for effective interprofessional working there is nothing obvious or taken for granted about who takes on the leadership role. While sometimes leadership will be prescribed by a particular role, there is no logical reason why position in a hierarchy should determine leadership. In some instances it does indeed come with the territory (so to speak), so the ECC in Chapter 2 is clear that his 'role . . . in an emergency department is to oversee the management of all the patients by all the staff', and he obviously understands this as a leadership role. Further this leadership role is extended into emergency situations outside the hospital environment, although this consultant recognizes the delicate negotiation required between the different emergency services where lines of 'being-in-charge' may converge:

> you are with people you have never met before and have to form teams in a very short space of time . . . How do you get things done effectively in a way that allows everyone to contribute, using their skills in a way that doesn't undermine the whole process of care?

The default position of this consultant seems to be one in which he anticipates that he and the other professionals he works with will satisfy the willingness condition and the trust condition. Indeed, this anticipation, which seems likely to generate a climate of trust between professionals, may be the key to meeting the leadership condition. As the obstetric consultant(2) in Chapter 4 notes:

> the midwives know far more than you guys [junior doctors] know, and you must respect them and defer to them, they're professionals in their own right.

There are many types of situations in which leadership need not be determined by hierarchical position, although one of the dangers of this is that no one may take responsibility for taking charge. This can be a problem when, as the physiotherapist in Chapter 2 notes, 'someone else thinks someone else is doing it and yes, it really impacts on service delivery'. This is something Florence Nightingale understood when she wrote:

> let whoever is in charge keep this simple question in her head (*not*, how can I always do this right thing myself, but) how can I provide for this right thing to be always done?
>
> (Nightingale 1980 [1859]:30)

This sentiment is reflected by the ECC in Chapter 2:

> if the medical staff are busy, the nursing staff take blood. It doesn't really matter, does it? What is important is that somebody does it and it fits into the overall workload of the department.

Summary

Three conditions related to ethics and values have been identified in this chapter as necessary for effective interprofessional practice. I have indicated that while there are personal characteristics that those who wish to engage with interprofessional practice should strive to develop (the willingness and the trust conditions), structural and institutional factors can either hinder or enable the development of these personal attributes. As the ECC in Chapter 2 notes, 'It requires a certain type of individual to work well in teams'; the type of individual he appears to have in mind is one who has the necessary skills for their particular professional role; who is willing to subsume personal and professional aspirations for the benefit of the goals of the team; who has sufficient professional wisdom to recognize the value of trusting other professionals to make valuable contributions to the team; and who can not only exhibit appropriate leadership skills when the need arises but also understand that hierarchal position does not necessarily equate with effective leadership qualities. It seems to me that each of the conditions are more easily met by those professionals who are sufficiently comfortable with the uncertainties that work with clients and patients inevitably involves to recognize that they cannot ever provide all the services that any one patient or client requires. This realization requires a certain humility (a character trait often dismissed as a weakness and inappropriate in the hard-nosed environment of modern social and health care), together with an openness about who should be doing what to (or with) whom, and a willingness to admit that one does not know everything.

Key points

■ Three conditions for effective interprofessional working are proposed; the conditions of willingness, trust and leadership.

■ The supposed common value set of different social and health care groups can be undermined by specific professional perspectives. This is further compounded by personal and professional differences in emphasis in regard to act- or agent-based ethics.

■ Individual practitioners may be encouraged or discouraged in their pursuit of approximating the three conditions by personal, professional and structural influences.

References

AIMS (2004) The case of Beatrice Carla. *AIMS Journal* 16(1):22.

Aristotle (1953 edn) *The Nichomachean Ethics*. Harmondsworth:Penguin.

Beauchamp T, Childress T (2001) *Principles of Biomedical Ethics* (5th edn) Oxford:Oxford University Press.

Couturier Y, Gagnon D, Carrier S, Etheridge F (2008) The interdisciplinary condition of work in relational professions of the health and social care field: a theoretical standpoint. *Journal of Interprofessional Care* 22:341–51.

GMC (2006) *Good Medical Practice*. London:General Medical Council.

GSCC (2002) *Code of Practice for Social Care Workers and Employers*. London:General Social Care Council.

HM Government (2008) *Information Sharing: Guidance for Practitioners and Managers*. Annesley:Department for Children, Schools and Families.

HPC (2008) *Standards of Conduct, Performance and Ethics.* London:Health Professions Council.

Hursthouse R (1997) Virtue ethics and abortion. In: Statman D (ed) (1997) *Virtue Ethics: A Critical Reader.* Edinburgh:Edinburgh University Press,227–44.

Irvine R, Kerridge I, McPhee J, Freeman S (2002) Interprofessionalism and ethics: consensus or clash of cultures? *Journal of Interprofessional Care* 16:199–210.

Kvarnstrom S (2008) Difficulties in collaboration: a critical incident study of interprofessional health care teamwork. *Journal of Interprofessional Care* 22:191–203.

Laurance J (1999) Midwives fear 'backlash' over natural births. *Independent* 10 May:9.

MacIntyre A (1985) *After Virtue: A Study in Moral Theory.* London:Duckworth.

Nightingale F (1980) *Notes on Nursing: What It Is and What It Is Not.* Edinburgh:Churchill Livingstone. (First published 1859 by Harrison & Sons, London).

NMC (2004) *Nursing and Midwifery Council (Midwives) Rules 2004.* London:Nursing and Midwifery Council.

NMC (2008) *The NMC Code of Professional Conduct: Standards for Conduct, Performance and Ethics.* London: Nursing and Midwifery Council.

O'Neill O (2002) *A Question of Trust: The BBC Reith Lectures 2002.* Cambridge:Cambridge University Press.

Pecukonis E, Doyle O, Bliss DL (2008) Reducing barriers to interprofessional training: promoting interprofessional cultural competence. *Journal of Interprofessional Care* 22:417–28.

Potter NN (2002) *How Can I Be Trusted? A Virtue Theory of Trustworthiness.* Lanham, MD:Rowman & Littlefield.

Pullon S (2008) Competence, respect and trust: key features of successful interprofessional nurse–doctor relationships. *Journal of Interprofessional Care* 22:133–47.

Race P (2006) *The Lecturer's Toolkit.* (3rd edn) London:Routledge.

Sellman D (2000) Alasdair MacIntyre and the professional practice of nursing. *Nursing Philosophy* 1:26–33.

Sellman D (2003) Open-mindedness: a virtue for professional practice. *Nursing Philosophy* 4:17–24.

Sellman D (2006) The importance of being trustworthy. *Nursing Ethics* 13:105–15.

Sellman D (2007) Trusting patients, trusting nurses. *Nursing Philosophy* 8:28–36.

Sockett H (1993) *The Moral Base for Teacher Professionalism.* New York:Teachers College Press.

Service Users, Carers and Issues for Collaborative Practice

Judith Thomas

Introduction

Health and social care services exist in order to provide services to people who need them. Interprofessional working is about providing better services, but what does this mean? Who is constructing what is good or better? Services are experiencing a major transformation not only in relation to the emphasis on collaborative working, but also in relation to the way in which the people who use these services and those in caring roles expect to be involved in decisions about care, treatment and service development at personal and organizational levels. Legislation and policies, for example those identified in the introduction to this book, increasingly require professionals to work in partnership with people who use services and the family members, neighbours and others who are also involved in their care.

Part I refers to people receiving services as patients, clients, service users, prisoners, consumers, carers, parents and mothers, but interestingly not fathers, so this chapter will start by considering the meanings that underpin some of these terms. It will then examine some Part I material to consider how the people who access the services discussed are viewed and positioned. This analysis will then be considered in relation to some of the literature and research on participation and empowerment. For example, in his consideration of multiprofessional teams, Payne (2000) suggests that the emphasis on relationships between the professionals in such teams can detract from the involvement and empowerment of the people who use these services.

Scrutiny of material in Part I identified different levels of service user involvement, participation and control. It should be remembered that the material in Part I is extracted from various studies and interviews. Some of those interviewed were asked specifically about user or carer involvement, whereas others were not. The excerpts were selected from much longer interviews in order to demonstrate the range of topics covered in this book. Some of the interviewees explicitly link their comments to their perception of the experience of the people at the receiving end of their interventions. In other cases the user is less visible. Consequently it cannot be assumed that the extracts used in Part I typify the attitudes of professionals interviewed. Despite these limitations an analysis of the data raises some fundamental but challenging issues to critique and consequently provides insights to inform and develop more inclusive collaborative practice.

We all have multiple identities. One service user organization suggests that 'the term "service user" can be used to restrict your identity as if all you are is a passive recipient of health and welfare services' (Shaping Our Lives National User Network 2003, cited in Warren 2007:8). I write as someone who, at times, has been a passive recipient of services. I construct myself, at my peril, as a long-distance 'carer' to my fiercely independent mother who lives in sheltered housing. I witness her 'rage against the dying of the light' (Thomas 1952) as, at the age of 92, she is forced to use services she would rather be providing. My early learning of interprofessional working was as the daughter of a pharmacist witnessing collaboration between him, district nurses and GPs, who would regularly call in to his dispensary. I have worked as a social worker, so experienced many of the benefits and frustrations of interprofessional working articulated in Part I, and now my identity includes that of an academic who has the privilege of working alongside many people who describe themselves as 'experts by experience' of using health and social care services.

As already noted, various terms or labels are used to describe us when we need to access services. These labels present two related challenges, one being to consider the implications of the labels and the other to decide on what terms to use in this chapter. The power inherent in the way language is used and discourses constructed is well established by authors such as Foucault (2000) and Bourdieu (1997) and by those writing about the professions such as Payne (2002) and Heffernan (2006). Any term used is likely to be problematic. The meanings of 'patient', as someone who is receiving treatment from health professionals and also as someone who waits, immediately implies a passivity. The term 'client' was popular in the 1970s and 1980s to describe people who received social work services. It was criticized for its implication that those using care services were similar to the 'clients' of solicitors or accountants or banks; but in the latter case people have choices about who they engage with and the term therefore does not take into account that some 'clients' prefer not to be receiving health and social care services, and those who do have little or no choice in the personnel providing the service. Heffernan (2006:140) considers 'its overtones of professionalism and expertise were thought to hold social control over those who used social care services'. The term 'service user' gained popularity in the 1990s but, with the new millennium, critiques of this term emerged. Heffernan considers its association with 'New Public Management', noting how the label can be a tool for restricting the population eligible to use particular services. She also highlights the negative connotations of users in relation to illegal 'drug users' and the common interpretation of 'user' as someone who exploits others. Referring to people as 'consumers' is also problematic as, like 'client', the term is used in commercial services and has the implication that, similar to 'patient' and 'user', it can be constructed as passive takers or people who consume services. Asking people what their preferred term is may resolve the problem at an individual level but research, cited in Heffernan (2006), illustrates that there is no consensus around terminology so therefore it is not possible to find a generic label that is acceptable to everyone. Consequently in this chapter, as far as possible, I have avoided using labels and talked about 'people'. However, some terms are used occasionally, but in doing this I acknowledge the problematic nature of any label and urge the reader to be mindful of the wider debates on this topic.

ACTIVITY

Think about some of your experiences of using services – how do these inform the way you interact as a professional?

What is your view of the different terms?

When do you think of yourself as a patient, client or service user?

There are various ways of conceptualizing service user and carer participation. The notion of a 'ladder of participation' was developed by Arnstein in 1969. The ladder starts on the lower rungs with non-participation, identified as manipulation and therapy, then moves on to tokenism, where people are informed and consulted, but essentially placated. Positions towards the top of the ladder are characterized by partnership, delegated power and citizen control. Arnstein's ladder has informed other work on participation; for example at organizational level, Hart (1997) has adapted it and developed the ladder to apply it to children's services while Nocon and Qureshi (1998) relate it to adult community services and Hoyes *et al.* (1993) make connections at individual levels of participation. Critiques of Arnstein's ladder identify problems with seeing participation in this hierarchical way. Kirby *et al.* (2003) highlight the complexity of different situations, contexts, tasks, the nature of the decisions being made, the individual's abilities and preferences, and the organizational culture. The material in Part I considered in the next section illustrates the range of attitudes to participation and the complexity of this notion.

People or objects?

While professionals may have moved on from referring to people as 'the appendix in bed six' there are examples of the location rather than the person being referred to. The children's nurse in Chapter 2 notes, 'They will walk straight to the trolley or they will walk to a bed', while the obstetric consultant in Chapter 4 refers to 'all the rooms' rather than the people in them. There are also examples of people being reduced to objects to which things are done:

> Like if it was chest pain, obviously we'd do observations, ECG [electrocardiogram] all that sort of thing, bloods.
>
> Adult nurse(2), Chapter 2

There is a sense that the taking of blood is displaced from the person as if it was being taken from a shelf rather than a living being. While there may be benefits from the flexibility of the medical or the nursing team being able to provide this service, as described by the emergency care consultant (ECC) in Chapter 2, it is also problematic. 'Taking blood' may be a routine procedure for the practitioners, but it is not necessarily seen in this way by the people whose blood it is or by the parents of a newborn baby, as this quote illustrates:

> We weren't really keen on the blood glucose tests . . . but I'm not sure if we really objected to them doing them over and over again how difficult it would have been to get that through to them.
>
> Service user(4), Chapter 4

The degree of intervention varied between settings working in the same service area as noted in the quote that follows. This conveys some of the complexity referred to by Kirby *et al.* (2003) that, while in some circumstances partnership working may be curtailed by the level of urgency or seriousness of a situation, this cannot be assumed and practices are dictated by the organizational culture:

> The paediatricians are . . . very hot on doing lots of observations and things on babies, and weighing babies, and doing all these things which I just wasn't used to when I came here [to the unit].
>
> Community midwife(3), Chapter 4

Other examples of viewing people as objects can be seen in obstetric consultant(2)'s comment in Chapter 4 about who can 'get the women delivered'. Interestingly, when the interviewees are talking about the management of a task their objectifying of people is much more pronounced than when they are discussing care or treatment. This is illustrated by the way in which the same consultant talks about the benefits of the contributions of different professionals who all 'want as many healthy women and healthy babies as possible'.

ACTIVITY

Can you think of any occasions when you were anxious about a procedure that the professionals saw as being 'routine'?

Another example of collaborative working as a mechanism to move people through can be seen in this quote from a consultant geriatrician in Chapter 2:

> I think we work very hard as a team to keep people moving through.

In this scenario the social worker raises her concerns, possibly linked to reservations about how much the person to be 'moved through' has had a voice in the decision:

> they'll find a vacancy at a nursing home for a particular person still in hospital. But we know it is completely inappropriate, but they might have gone ahead and told the family and it is quite difficult to undo all that.
>
> Social worker(2), Chapter 2

While these examples illustrate the advantages of flexibility they also highlight the problem of creating or maintaining a culture of different professionals constructing people as subjects to be 'done to', 'moved on', 'moved through' or 'delivered'. The potential for different members of the team providing checks and balances to have a mitigating effect on this culture is illustrated by the social worker's comments in the example above. It also provides scope for working more collaboratively with the people who need services, so supporting the breakdown of traditional professional boundaries. This can be seen by the contrasting examples in Chapters 4 and 2. The senior midwife in Chapter 4 refers to how she

> had to call a consultant over the head of a registrar and say, 'I'm not happy with your decision, if you're not prepared to discuss it with me I'm going to call the consultant.'

This situation is presented as a difference of opinion between the registrar and the midwife with the consultant acting as referee; the perspectives of the mother and her partner seem to be absent. In contrast, the children's nurse in Chapter 2 capitalizes on the mother's need for information to challenge an orthopaedic doctor on the way s/he communicates with other members of the team, in the process drawing attention to the impact of the lack of communication on the family:

> 'Right, so you need to either come back and write in the notes or come and communicate with somebody regarding this because we have now got a mother coming in to the nurses' station asking what's going on; and do we know what's going on? No, because you haven't told us, so now I'm bothering you and bleeping your pager to tell me what's going on.'

Professionals are aware of their responsibility to work collaboratively whilst ensuring that people get an appropriate service, as shown by the children's nurse in the example above. Professionals are also aware of the need to advocate and support the wishes of people for particular courses of action, as illustrated in the quotes below:

> We spend a lot of time trying to be the patients' advocate. There was a lot of messing around with certain types of patient . . . Failed paperwork, people being sent out too early and bouncing back in too readily. Failures getting in, failures getting out. Patients not knowing what was happening . . . Admissions cancelled, notes lost and the doctor's letter getting lost.
>
> GP, Chapter 1

> I know she [the midwife] had tried to lobby to allow us to go home straight after the baby was born.
>
> Service user(4), Chapter 4

ACTIVITY

Why is the idea of advocacy important in health and social care? Can you identify any advocacy services in your area of work?

Information giving, consultation and consent

Professionals and service users offer interesting perspectives on the extent to which even the most basic levels of participation, such as the right to information, were met. The GP in Chapter 1 offers a vivid illustration of how professionals assume a level of knowledge or don't ensure the person has understood the medical procedure or treatment:

> Sometimes they would come in into the surgery weeks later with ECG [electrocardiograph] leads still on their chests, patients thinking it was part of treatment to have these plastic things stuck to them.

Two of the women in Chapter 4 make interesting observations about consultation and informed consent:

> they then explained to me why it would be a great thing, in fact they weren't really explaining to me why it would be a great thing if I got induced, they were explaining to me why they were going to induce me, essentially.
>
> Service user(3)

Service user(3) also comments on her feelings of intimidation by the postures and positions adopted by the professionals: 'they were stood very close, stood up as well, I was sitting down'. She goes on to say:

> it was very brusque and businesslike and, 'Let's get on with the arrangements' [clicks fingers] rather than taking me through benefits, risks, alternatives maybe, a bit more explanation as to why it would be necessary, do I have any questions.

Another woman comments on her perception of the obstetric registrar who:

> just wasn't communicative and wasn't able to understand that we might not be keen on having a scan or doing a test or doing this and that, staying in hospital, he just seemed to think that whatever he suggested ought to be exactly what we did.
>
> Service user(4)

Service user(4) appreciates the role other members of the team play in ensuring they have understood treatments and the value of someone taking time to explain things in more detail:

> the midwife was useful when she came back after he'd gone . . . she was quite good at sitting down and explaining what she thought was going on, so it was good and bad . . . she was very supportive.

The senior registrar working in paediatrics (SRP) in Chapter 3 emphasizes the importance of communication and consultation with children:

> I always treat children as I would treat an adult, although the words you use sometimes are different. The longer that a child has been in the system, the more generally they understand . . . So they've had four years of treatment and they're on their second bone-marrow transplant; you should listen to them, if they say, 'Listen, I'm not sure I want to do this again' . . . they would have a very good understanding . . . and the parents equally would have a very good understanding, and you could have a much more educated discussion with them.

Whose patient is it, anyway?

The material in Part I raises interesting issues on the notion of ownership and how this can be constructed. This comment by the GP in Chapter 1 illustrates how professionals can view people as belonging to them:

District nurses were the most interwoven with our practice, they see our patients all time.

As well as potentially indicating the ownership of the person as belonging with a professional in this instance, and in the example that follows, the possessive pronoun relates to the doctor, rather than the nurse:

'No, this is who you need to talk to, they are looking after your patient.'

Children's nurse, Chapter 2

The use of 'my' or 'our' also occurs frequently in relation to membership of a team, for example, 'our social workers'. There are examples of users of services referring to the professionals they work with in the same way, as in the service user in Chapter 5 talking about 'My social worker'. While it could be argued that the term is unproblematic, as it is used in a benign way by both professionals and service users, this does not take account of the power differences between professionals and users or how it can contribute to the latter feeling disempowered, as expressed in this example:

it was almost like, 'You're ours now, we can do what we like and that's it, you're here', almost, rather than working with, you know, somebody who's clearly heavily pregnant, clearly quite upset.

Service user(3), Chapter 4

The concerns of this woman resonate with those of SRP in Chapter 3 who comments on the attitude adopted by a colleague who

kept describing information she was giving, she wants the patient apparently to fit in with our agenda, on the basis that if you do as we tell you, you'll get better.

In Chapter 2, ECC highlights the need for empowerment in teamworking:

People aren't empowered to speak up, people aren't being used in a functioning team.

This consultant shows an awareness of other aspects of power, highlighting how people can feel threatened when it is questioned:

They feel it undermines their power or their self-esteem...that it will undermine status and position.

The same consultant highlights the advantages of teamwork in terms of safe care:

When you have multiple people involved in a single process it gives you multiple checks and balances in a system and it stops people doing something very abnormal.

As opposed to:

One person, thinking in an illogical way, not thinking very clearly in a situation, if they have a lot of power they can make a lot of mistakes.

ECC, Chapter 2

Mental health nursing student(2) in Chapter 5 raises her concerns about the controlling nature of the consultant at a ward round:

I don't know why she was controlling, but she was controlling the course of the meeting and she had to prompt everyone, everyone's opinions about each service user and go through one to the other.

It is not clear, from the student's account, whether service users were part of these discussions. Given the controlling way in which the meeting was chaired it is difficult to see how, even if they were able to put forward their views or preferences, service users would be able to have any real influence on plans or decisions about their treatment. Judging from the conclusion reached by a forensic service user-led research study, referred to in Chapter 5, there are services where shared planning and working with service users is a long way off:

it became very apparent that service users often fear and second-guess what is being said about them in ward rounds, case conferences handovers, etcetera, and what records are being constructed about them.

In this instance, despite staff views of teamworking being limited, it adds an additional dimension to service users' perceptions of power as they

saw the staff as very united in their practice, albeit in a rather negative way.

Service user perspectives, Chapter 5

====== **ACTIVITY** ======

Think of an occasion when you have experienced someone as being controlling. What behaviour did he or she exhibit?

Now identify an occasion when you were aware of a shift in power – what happened to enable this?

Moving from consultation, to involvement, to greater user control

The introduction of direct payments (Great Britain 1996) allows people to be more in control of their own care and to 'buy in' services. This creates a fundamental shift in the balance of power between those who need services and professionals. Service user(1)'s account in Chapter 3 shows she has some control and influence over her care. It is 'mutually agreed' between her and the social worker when another practitioner is needed and the service user is the 'employer' who 'hires and fires'. Despite this shift the initial assessment is undertaken by a professional, although all the guidance for the *Single Assessment Process* (DH 2002) does require this to be done in 'partnership'. In the same chapter the carer's story illustrates the challenges of working in partnership, drawing attention to the difference between assuming and listening or giving her mother time to 'speak in her own language', that is, really communicating rather than speaking on another person's behalf. The carer emphasizes the importance of 'dignity and respect, listening to people and not being too prescriptive'. The notion of 'true user involvement' is also articulated by the health visitor quoted in this chapter. The value of a co-ordinated holistic assessment process and the benefits of not having to give the same information to different people are also discussed, so confirming the importance to users of communication, shared record-keeping and collaboration.

The individual narratives of service users already discussed illustrate their variable experiences of consultation and involvement in their treatment. Their narratives also show the need for users and carers to take more control, not least for their own safety. Service user(1) 'almost choked in bed' following a rushed service so chose to sit up the following night rather than take this risk again. Service user(2) in Chapter 4 also needed to be vigilant to ensure she received treatment that was meant to be a standard procedure agreed under NICE (National Institute for Clinical Excellence) guidelines.

Part I prompts discussion of consultation at more of a structural and organizational level as well as in relation to individuals. The organization that provides a brokerage service to which Service user(1) in Chapter 3 refers is one of many user organizations that also lobby for more influence in the design and delivery of services. They also work to promote a real, rather than tokenistic, philosophy of users and carers having more control and influence on services, for example, through their websites Shaping our Lives (www.shapingourlives.org.uk/) and the Princess Royal Trust for Carers (www.carers.org/). As such they are illustrations of positions on the higher rungs of Arnstein's (1969) ladder of participation. The reflections of the voluntary-sector personnel that follow illuminate some of the complexity and tensions associated with meaningful participation, developing inclusive management structures and the construction of a professional.

In Chapter 3 the community development worker describes how the starting point for the development of services was based on a survey of what people 'needed and wanted'. She identifies how government directives do not necessarily make for 'meaningful consultation' and considers the strategies she employs to ensure she is not only representing the views of the community but also creating changes in policy. The community development worker's strategies include challenging by checking out meanings and trying to 'couch things in terms of constructive suggestions'. She anticipates how her suggestions may be being received, using phrases like 'you must be sick of the sound of my voice by now', giving the message that she is self-aware and sensitive to others while conveying firmness of purpose and her responsibility to present the views of the community, despite the fact that these challenge the status quo. Her comments about the mechanisms of meetings illustrate the persistence needed to bring about change in structures and services to make them more consistent with the needs of the community:

> I don't know that it's anything more than meetings and paper. The usual thing, you get reports, you read reports, you underline things in red, you go to meetings, raise questions, and those get minuted, in however legible or illegible a form, and then on to the next thing.

The need for persistence can also be seen in the accounts of the service users, for example Service user(1)'s description in Chapter 3 of following through concerns about the services she received. This persistence takes time, energy and resources, themes that are echoed in the same chapter by the manager of a large voluntary agency (MLVA), as she reflects on the gap between government policies and the reality on the ground.

The philosophy behind the development of Sure Start services promoted partnership between different disciplines and the people for whom services were being provided. The manager distinguishes between 'user control rather than just user involvement' and goes on to describe 'capacity building'. She articulates a range of structures that supported parents having greater power. For example, at structural level, where parents 'made up half of the management board', and parents who were employed or worked as volunteers, through to working in partnership with individual parents and children, for example, on a drop-in basis to help with speech and language development. Her experiences in this setting led her to comment that

> Different professional groups have very different understanding, experiences and attitudes around participation and there can be tensions around this.

Kirby *et al.* (2003) identify the tensions and challenges of moving through the different levels of participation. The problem of resource constraints, notably around the time involved in consultation and short-term funding, are evident in the narratives in Chapter 3:

> you see wonderful things started . . . you know they have done so much good, so many people wanted them and now they've just disappeared again . . . often you can't do enough long enough.
>
> Community development worker

Another challenge relates to confidentiality and accountability, noted by the GP in Chapter 1 when discussing issues related to patient's rights and protection:

]doctors are worried about confidentiality, there are huge issues . . . what can I tell the social worker, I know there is a risk here . . . but what ball will it start rolling?

Also in relation to relationships between professionals, users and carers:

We are much more aware of who is caring for who; and patient confidentiality is important here.

The MLVA in Chapter 3 outlines different strategies used to address confidentiality at organization and policy level with 'clear guidelines on how to make referrals' and how these dilemmas can be used as the basis for mutual learning in an interdisciplinary context:

we had a system where at inter-agency team meetings people took it in turns to talk about their roles, and it was open to anyone working or funded by Sure Start to participate. Different professions would take the agenda for half an hour and share what they thought others needed to know about their service and interprofessional or inter-agency dilemmas and issues. As a lot of the para-professionals were local parents, this was a really good opportunity for capacity building.

There is a stark contrast between the practices in the Sure Start setting and the unit described in Chapter 5:

the term [interprofessional] implicitly suggests that service users do not have a real part to play in its collaborative procedure. Their only contribution is as consumers that might give their opinion about the services professionals provide, which regulate patients' behaviour within a secure (prison-like) environment.

Discussion and conclusions

So what conclusions can be drawn about the extent to which users of services and the carers are central to interprofessional working? Clearly there is a long way to go in some instances, as exemplified by the practices in the forensic unit and the way in which professionals set the agenda and determine treatments. There is little reference to the concerns or wishes of the people they are treating with whom, according to their own professional codes and national service frameworks, they should be working in partnership.

Central to participation is the notion of empowerment, a term that is used more often than it is defined and one that Faulkner (2001) identifies is interpreted in various ways. Faulkner's study of health care settings analyses behaviours that have the effect of being empowering or disempowering. Within his discussion he identifies empowering acts such as staff providing information relating to future care options, respecting patients' choices and seeking patients' permission prior to conducting tasks. Examples of these behaviours were highlighted in relation to midwives' interventions with service users (3) and (4) and in the concern of the SRP to work with families.

Faulkner (2001) also outlines acts that disempowered people. These included 'dismissing patients' complaints', adopting 'dominant postures when talking to patients' and 'preventing patients from making decisions about their planned care'. Examples of these disempowering actions are apparent in the section relating to 'Information giving, consultation or consent' above, such as in the case of the service user raising concerns relating to treatments not being provided, people feeling that procedures were imposed, and feeling intimidated by the stance adopted by the professionals, demonstrated explicitly by their physical position and implicitly in their attitude.

Kirby *et al.*'s (2003) comment on the complexity of participation and the interaction between the capacity of individuals to make choices and the impact of the organization are essential to bear in mind when thinking of the range of services provided in health and social care. The limitations of the material in Part I make it difficult to draw any firm conclusions about how these factors interact. Professionals may perceive users and carers with a stronger voice as being in conflict with their understanding of their professional accountability and be concerned about increased risks to the users, litigation or to wider society, as in the case of the forensic science unit. However, as the studies, for example those referred to in Godin (2006), show, perceptions of risk are not just determined by the setting or the nature of the person's condition.

ACTIVITY

What factors can you identify that limit participation? What can be done to overcome them?

The greater emphasis on teamworking does provide staff with the basis on which to challenge these more dominant behaviours and traditional hierarchies, as demonstrated by the children's nurse's assertive behaviour with medical personnel. Her concern to work in a more empowering way with the mother by ensuring that she is provided with basic details of treatment is an example of the nurse using the power of her position to ensure a better service. The importance of modelling empowering approaches in relation to teamworking is evident in the emergency care consultant's comments relating to the empowerment of team members. This is a crucial basis for moving towards the position advocated by Payne (2000), Barton (2003) and Beresford (2007), with the locus of control being in the domain of users and carers, rather than automatically with the professionals.

There are examples of services being developed and delivered with and for users and attempts to put them at the 'heart of the service' (DH 1998). However, policy changes, such as direct payments, that set the scene for users to have more control over their lives, also come with challenges and responsibilities, as Service user(1) indicates. So unless there is more emphasis and awareness generally of the rights of people using services, the greater the challenge will be in making them work. In the examples from Sure Start and the voluntary (third) sector we can see the attention to detail, the attitudinal change required of staff and the organizational philosophy that is required to move beyond what Braye (2000:19) crystallizes as the 'illusion of participation'.

Summary

In this chapter, the author initially noted the problematic nature of many terms applied to people using health or social care services. Hence it behoves professionals to be mindful of the wider debates on this topic. The chapter then discusses ways in which people who access services are viewed and positioned in relation to some of the literature and research on participation and empowerment. Conclusions drawn include the following:

■ The emphasis on relationships between different professionals in collaborative working can detract from the involvement and empowerment of the people who use services as identified by Payne (2000).

■ A variety of terms are used to describe people who access health and social care services and there is no consensus about terminology.

■ Recent developments in policy and legislation promote the need for professionals to develop ways of working collaboratively with service users and carers.

■ Professionals need to challenge each other to ensure that service users and carers are part of the team and that working practices are developed in order to support this.

■ Moving from user participation to user control requires us to analyse different levels of participation and to consider how power operates within teams and organizations.

References

Arnstein S (1969) A ladder of citizen participation in the USA. *Journal of the American Institute of Planners* 35(4):216–24.

Barton C (2003) Allies and enemies: the service user as care co-ordinator. In: Weinstein J, Whittington C, Leiba T (eds) *Collaboration in Social Work Practice*. London:Jessica Kingsley, 103–20.

Beresford P (2007) *The Changing Roles and Tasks of Social Work: From Service Users' Perspectives: A literature-informed discussion paper.* Shaping Our Lives National User Network www.shapingourlives.org.uk/ (Accessed1.05.2009).

Bourdieu P (1997) *Language and Symbolic Power.* Oxford:Blackwell.

Braye S (2000) Participation and involvement in social care: an overview. In: Kempshall H, Littlechild R (eds) *User Involvement and Participation in Social Care: Research Informing Practice.* London:Jessica Kingsley, 9–28.

DH (1998) *Modernising Social Services: Promoting Independence, Improving Protection, Raising Standards.* London:The Stationery Office.

DH (2002) *Single Assessment Process.* London:Department of Health.

Faulkner M (2001) Models of empowerment and disempowerment. *NT research* 6(6):936–48.

Foucault M (2000) *Power*, ed. James D. Faubion. New York:The New Press.

Godin P (ed) (2006) *Risk and Nursing Practice.* Basingstoke:Palgrave Macmillan.

Great Britain (1996) *Community Care (Direct Payments Act).* London:Her Majesty's Stationery Office.

Hart R (1997) *Children's Participation: The Theory and Practice of Involving Young Citizens in Community Development and Environmental Care.* London:Earthscan.

Heffernan K (2006) Social work, new public management and the language of 'service user'. *British Journal of Social Work* 36:139–47.

Hoyes L, Jeffers S, Lart R, Means R, Taylor M (1993) *User Empowerment and the Reform of Community Care: A Study of Early Implementation in Four Localities.* Bristol:SAUS Publications, University of Bristol.

Kirby P, Lanyon C, Cronin K, Sinclair R (2003) *Building a Culture of Participation. Involving Children and young People in Policy, Service Planning, Delivery and Evaluation. Research Report.* London:Department for Education and Skills.

Nocon A, Qureshi H (1998) *Outcomes of Community Care for Users and Carers: A Social Services Perspective.* Buckingham:Open University Press.

Payne M (2000) *Teamwork in Multiprofessional Care.* Basingstoke:Palgrave Macmillan.

Payne M (2002) The role and achievements of a professional association in the later twentieth century: the British association of social workers 1970–2000. *British Journal of Social Work* 32:969–95.

Shaping Our Lives National User Network (2003) www.shapingourlives.org.uk/.

Thomas D (1952) Do Not Go Gentle Into That Good Night. In: *The Poems of Dylan Thomas.* New York:New Directions.

Warren J (2007) *Service User and Carer Participation in Social Work.* Exeter:Learning Matters.

Conclusions and Future Directions

Judith Thomas

Introduction

The wealth of material and different perspectives in this book provide a unique overview of professional, service user and academic perspectives. The challenge now is to identify how these different voices can shape the future of health and social care alongside emerging policy, legislation and other developments.

Among other themes, most chapters make some reference to power, particularly in relation to the medical profession (notably Pollard in Chapter 9) and the relationships between service users and professionals (notably Thomas in Chapter 12). This chapter will look at the shifting nature of power and how members of interprofessional teams, including service users, can use their power constructively. This analysis will be linked to Oliver and Keeping's (Chapter 7) discussion of identities being in a 'state of flux' and Miers's consideration of new models of professionalism (Chapter 8). It will identify how the recent legislation and policies, identified by Pollard in the introductory chapter, support more power sharing and will also consider some of the associated challenges outlined in Harle *et al.'s* analysis of organizational complexity (Chapter 10). This discussion will pick up on some of the contradictions in policies, such as expectations around the 'lead professional' and dilemmas relating to information sharing. Following on from this, the chapter will highlight how critical reflection is needed for effective implementation of policy and legislation where interprofessional working is promoted.

The focus of the book is on the application and development of theory to inform, analyse and evaluate interprofessional working. This chapter will connect this to the 'willingness condition' outlined by Sellman (Chapter 11) and argue that the commitment to 'do whatever is required to contribute to effective teamworking' (Sellman *ibid.*) includes developing theoretical frameworks to deepen understanding and to inform new practices. This will lead into a discussion of the learning theories Miers discusses (Chapter 6), in particular connecting with Wenger's 'communities of practice' (1998). The potential of 'communities of practice' to enhance the quality of care will be considered, and within these the need for different perspectives and conflicts to be used creatively in order to provide the complex range of services that may be needed. The chapter includes recommendations for the education of existing and emerging professionals and concludes with further suggestions for development in relation to practice, policy and theory.

Individual interpersonal level of interprofessional working

Part II of this book analyses the different factors that impact on interprofessional working. At the interpersonal level Oliver and Keeping identify how our individual defence mechanisms may emerge in working relationships (Chapter 7). They consider how the formation of our identities influences our capacity to work with others. However, when considering the influence of our early lives there will also be learnt behaviours that facilitate our ability to collaborate, such as participating in teams, clubs and societies. It may be that one of the barriers to interprofessional working has been our preoccupation and identification with established ways of working and particular professional backgrounds. Consequently we have not appreciated or celebrated our own capacity to adapt and develop. Being more aware of the notion of shifting identities and our capacity to change, take on new roles and adapt to different situations, may help us embrace the changes necessary to provide more integrated services. The questions in the box below will help you think about the skills and qualities that may make you a good team player. Consulting other members of a team or group you belong to will provide you with additional insights and also can promote others to think about their own contribution as well as yours. The questions in the box below will help broaden your thinking about teamworking and help you focus on your contribution in a positive way.

=== **CONCLUDING ACTIVITY** ===

Thinking about teamworking

What experiences, outside your working life, do you have of teamworking?

What particular skills and qualities do you bring to these teams?

How do you demonstrate these skills and qualities in your work groups or teams?

What do other members of the team value about your contribution?

Research into the effectiveness of interprofessional education has identified the value of students from different disciplines learning together. Originally the concept was encapsulated as being 'with, from and about each other' (Centre For The Advancement Of Interprofessional Education (CAIPE) 1997). However, Hammick *et al.* (2009:9) reconstruct this as occurring 'when learners from two or more professions learn about, from and with each other'. This revised version prioritizes the need for students to learn about each other in order to go on to learn with and from each other. In Chapter 6 Miers explores a number of studies that consider the evidence relating to the value of interprofessional education. Miers notes that many studies about interprofessional learning are at post-qualifying level, but developing awareness, skills and understanding of what constitutes a good team and our own contribution to this process needs to be part of professional training. One of the debates has focused on the best time to introduce interprofessional learning and at what stage of professional development this is likely to be most effective. Anyone working in health and social care must be able to communicate effectively and work collaboratively with people who use services as well as those providing services and this has always been the case. Whilst we do need to consider the most effective ways of developing and enhancing collaborative working skills this needs to start at the beginning of people's professional careers. The voices in Part I and the chapter authors in Part II of the book illustrate that collaborative working is not an optional extra but the essence of professional practice, a view emphasized by Hammick *et al.* (2009).

Essential skills and values

The imperatives of person-centred agendas (DH 2009), protecting children (Laming 2003, 2009) and providing integrated care mean that the interpersonal skills of listening, clarifying, conveying information and negotiation are as important as the specialist technical skills and knowledge practitioners need. If we accept that professionals in health and social care need to work with other people, then part of that right to define oneself as a professional will encompass what Race (1993) constructs as 'conscious competence' moving into the 'unconscious competence' of working with other professionals as well as with service users or patients. We would not contemplate having a debate about whether the ability to communicate with a service user should be part of professional training, so why do we do it in relation to interprofessional working? Working collaboratively is now a requirement of all professionals and consequently being a professional includes being able to work interprofessionally, not as an optional extra but as a core skill. Hammick *et al.* (2009:8) construct this as 'being interprofessional' and highlight that in order to do this we need to draw on relevant knowledge, skills and values. The editors hope that insights from practitioners and service users in Part I and theoretical discussions in Part II have enhanced your knowledge base and given you some insight into the skills required; and that Chapter 11 by Sellman has deepened your understanding of values in the context of interprofessional working.

As health and social care professionals we not only have occupational standards that require collaborative working but, as Sellman argues, also have a moral and ethical responsibility to do so. Furthermore, Clark (2006) argues that students need to show an awareness of the system of values and beliefs that underpin their own practice whilst appreciating that other professionals 'may have committed to a different, but equally valid, perspective based on their own values and belief systems' (Hean *et al.* 2008). It would be naive to suggest that because we have an ethical responsibility to collaborate and appreciate the views of others we will necessarily always practise in this way. The way in which services are led, as we have seen in Parts I and II of this book, can enhance or constrain collaborative working, a point also identified in many other studies, including Garrett and Lodge (2008) and Ham (2009). Harle *et al.* in Chapter 10 discuss how leadership involves explicitly drawing in the views of others; but more than this it involves creating a climate or a culture that clearly facilitates participation in relation to service users and any one involved in their care.

Power and leadership

At this stage it may be helpful to take the discussion away from the individual practitioner or leader and to consider how the application of theories of power can assist our analysis of interprofessional working and user participation. The voices in Part I and the analysis in Part II tend to concentrate on power in relation to professional roles and associated status. The complex interaction between ascribed roles and other power issues relating to class, gender, race and age that occur in interprofessional encounters identified by, for example, Clarke *et al.* (2007), Loxley (1997) and Payne (2000) also needs to be acknowledged. Professionals need to recognize power imbalances at structural and societal levels in relation to, amongst other aspects, the historical status of different professionals and the impact of gendered roles. These issues are discussed by Miers in Chapter 8, Pollard in Chapter 9 and Harle *et al.* in Chapter 10. An understanding of the interaction between structural power, the power that others may see as being invested in particular professions and the legitimate use of one's own personal power is necessary in order to challenge existing hegemonies.

The analyses of power and empowerment by the above authors in Chapters 8 to 10, and by Thomas in Chapter 12, offer theoretical frameworks to consider and deconstruct power dynamics. These chapters highlight that changes in roles, teams, leadership and organization of services have the potential to lead to greater collaboration between professionals and service users. However, we need to think about what is needed for this potential to be realized. What is necessary to achieve a culture that facilitates collaborative working and the involvement of everyone? What might a leader or manager of an interprofessional team need to do? Clearly, as Mental health nursing student(2)'s example of the consultant at the meeting in Chapter 5 illustrates, being able to delegate is essential. It is also necessary to be able to recognize when, because of status and traditional hierarchies, leadership is assumed to rest with a particular person or profession. So as practitioners we need to take responsibility not to perpetuate assumptions about leadership inevitably resting with a particular person – whether due to age, gender or professional role – but also to recognize that different members of a team can lead on particular aspects. The activity in the box below will help you think further about leadership and relate it to some of the theories that have been suggested in Part II of the book.

─────────────── **CONCLUDING ACTIVITY** ───────────────

Analysing leadership and power

Think of a situation where you have assumed someone else would lead in a particular situation or a situation where it has been assumed that you would take the lead. Analyse why this may have been the case – think about this in relation to professional role, status, age, gender, ethnicity, professional qualification, expert knowledge.

Choose one of the chapters that discuss power and empowerment (Chapters 8, 9, 10 or 12) and review your experience using one of the theories suggested. Identify how, if you were faced with a similar situation again, you could address the power dynamics and challenge assumptions being made about leadership.

This exercise may have led you to consider that clarifying the leadership role may not be straightforward. Different practitioners may have responsibility for different aspects of leadership, and power may need to shift accordingly. Within this context, the power of the service user or carer must also be considered and professionals will need to develop ways of relinquishing their own power, so promoting the empowerment of service users and carers. There will be times where the ability of the service user to determine their treatment or the level of intervention may be constrained by their mental or physical condition or by the need to protect others. However, as legislation such as the *Children Act* (Great Britain 1989), the *Human Rights Act* (Great Britain 1998) and the *Mental Capacity Act* (Great Britain 2005) requires, practitioners have a duty to work in partnership to ensure the highest level of participation possible.

Authors such as Day (2006) and Barrett and Keeping (2005) draw on a range of research studies to stress the need for clarity of role, whether this be about leadership or any other role. Again this imperative is fraught with difficulty, not least because roles are changing and developing. In some cases this results from changes to legislation, as in the case of nurses prescribing or social workers becoming care managers. In other cases new roles are being developed to meet demand for services, such as health care workers being able to undertake certain procedures or to develop a particular expertise. Miers discusses other examples in Chapter 8. The call for clarity of role begs the question as to whether the practitioner role can always be clear. We have already seen that the notion of a fixed identity is problematic, so it may be more helpful to look for the ability to negotiate roles as appropriate in different situations and recognize that circumstances may mean that these may change in the light of need.

Organizational factors and conflict

In Chapter 10, Harle *et al.* outline the complexity of the organizational systems and structures, while in Chapter 9, Pollard discusses the tensions between medical and social models of working and the dominance of the medical model. These aspects, together with the conundrums about role, are likely to create conflicts and tensions. Miers in Chapter 6 and Warmington *et al.*'s (2004) review of literature concerning inter-agency working identify that the emphasis on collaboration has implications for the way in which conflicts may be dealt with:

> It is still often implied that the conflicts generated by inter-agency working must be denied and that the ideal work form involves the coalescing of expertise into compact and consensual communities of practice.
>
> (*ibid.*:38)

Consequently one of the dangers of romanticizing collaboration is that the potential for learning and the value of constructive conflict and disagreement will be lost, as also identified by Garrett and Lodge (2008) and Hammick *et al.* (2009).

'Communities of practice' have their critics as identified by Miers in Chapter 6. Also, Tennant (1997) raises concerns about their limited analysis of power relationships and their lack of accountability within formal accreditation systems. However, there are examples of communities of practice bringing people from different disciplines together in order to learn from difficult situations, for example, in relation to adult protection (Thomas and Spreadbury 2008). The fact that these communities meet away from the pressures of day-to-day delivery of services may make them a safer place to learn from situations where conflict has occurred. They merit further research into their effectiveness.

One of the issues raised by enquiries such as the report into the death of Victoria Climbié (Laming 2003) and the Kennedy Report (2001) into child deaths relating to heart surgery at the Bristol Royal Infirmary, was that professionals did not challenge each other, thereby avoiding the possibility of conflict. Had different perspectives been encouraged this could potentially have lead to different outcomes. Pollard (Chapter 9) and Thomas (Chapter 12) discuss the value of practitioners challenging each other and the benefits in terms of outcomes for service users. Warmington *et al.* (2004) draw on the work of Engeström *et al.* (1997) to identify the need to find tools for disagreement. They argue that practitioners must develop their awareness of the limitations and potential dangers of viewing collaboration as a conflict free zone. Here a reminder of some of the introductory literature on group work may be helpful. Tuckman and Jensen (1977) emphasize the importance of the 'storming stage' of group development. Belbin (1981) identified the value of the different roles necessary for effective teamworking, for example, the radical and unorthodox thinking of what he identifies as the 'plant' role.

Anne Oakley (1984:80) takes the view that 'without conflict life is dead and art impossible'. The danger of avoiding conflict and the creativity that can come as a result of working through it need to be recognized and celebrated. This creativity has the potential to meet some of the concerns of service users for whom:

> Success would mean people in the community who need support and their familiars and carers feeling empowered to come up with flexible solutions to meet their needs, individually or collectively. . . . People feel they have a life rather than a set of services.
>
> (TASC Programme Board 2008:2)

The questions in the box that follows will help you to consider conflict in interprofessional working.

===== **CONCLUDING ACTIVITY** =====

Thinking about conflict

Identify a report or investigation that has identified problems that have occurred in professional practice. Review the report and identify how any conflicts were dealt with. Were they openly acknowledged or avoided? Where conflict was avoided consider why this may have been the case.

Now think about your own practice. When did you last hear a colleague passionately argue for a particular course of action? What was the response of others? How were different views accommodated? In what ways was the service provided enhanced or compromised by the conflict? What did you learn from the conflict?

Communities of practice offer the opportunity to capture and develop practice wisdom or theory that evolves from practice. Other forms of organizational learning, whether created formally through education programmes or promoted as part of team culture through good leadership, also have the potential to contribute to the development of theory. Sellman explores the 'willingness condition' that needs to be present for collaborative working to be effective; this condition can be applied to the development of theory and policy. Here again the contribution of the user as part of the construction of knowledge needs to be recognized, as discussed in Chapter 5 (see Godin *et al.* 2007 for more detail) and by Harle *et al.* (Chapter 10). Thomas (Chapter 12) identifies that the level of participation of service users and carers within the interprofessional team varies from very limited, at best tokenistic involvement, to influencing not only decisions about their own care but also the development of services. As highlighted in various chapters, practitioners need to develop their understanding of participation. An increasing wealth of research reports and reviews are available that identify ways of supporting this process, for example, Beresford and Banfield (2006) Crawford *et al.* (2003), Doel *et al.* (2007), Fauth and Mahdon (2007) and Roulstone *et al.* (2006).

Policy and legislation

We have considered interprofessional working from an individual perspective and a local perspective in terms of the team and the organization, so let us now briefly consider the wider structure of policy and legislation that inform practice. There are some anomalies here as identified in Chapter 3, such as the problems created by policy documents that identify health visitors as the lead professional. A study by the Nuffield Trust (Ham 2009) of progress into the integration of health and social care services identified the tensions in the policy between co-operation and competition created by the way in which funding is allocated through pooled budgets and commissioning. Ham's review came to the conclusion that:

> The absence of a coherent health and social care reform narrative is likely to hinder the next stage of reform in both services and in partnership working.
>
> (Ham 2009:12)

Key points to emerge from that study highlighted the need for the focus to be on the service user and agencies negotiating and discussing what is needed, rather than emphasizing 'structures and organisational solutions' (*ibid.*:1). Legislation and policies identified in the introduction to this book, relating to services for children and adults, all enshrine the need for greater collaborative working. The problems associated with the way in which funding is allocated have been acknowledged. This concern is taken forward in *Working to Put People First* (DH 2009), with one of the strategic priorities identified as being 'Workforce remodelling and commissioning' (p50). The personalization agenda in that document promotes universal services that extend way beyond health and social care boundaries. This initiative calls for wider community services, transport and housing to work in an integrated way. The policy aims to promote early intervention and prevention. It supports principles of choice and control, together with supporting and valuing the engagement of all members of communities. Inevitably the success of all these initiatives will depend on policymakers and practitioners working with users of services in an informed way.

The ever-expanding resource of research reviews, policy papers and detailed guidance referred to in this book can support practitioners in navigating the complexities of interprofessional working. However, the implementation of protocols and imperatives requires creative thinking, practice wisdom and expertise acquired from the lived experiences of service users, carers, practitioners and managers. Laming (2009) promotes moving beyond just relying on guidance and policies by stressing the need for this to be combined with critical reflection. Despite the wealth of guidance, relating for example to information sharing, the need for dialogue and opportunities to deconstruct terminology to arrive at a shared understanding is consistently identified in research studies, for example, Bokhour (2006), Reder and Duncan (2003) and Richardson and Asthana (2006).

The NHS review of health care (DH 2008) expands the notion of accountability beyond that of the individual practitioner, to accountability for the quality of the overall outcomes achieved. It identifies that this 'means a new accountability' that 'is for the whole patient pathway – so clinicians must be partners as well as practitioners.' (*ibid.*:64). This directive makes professionals responsible not just for their own practice but gives them wider accountability for the work of the team and the service provided. The paper emphasizes this developed notion of accountability by stressing that 'All the different parts of the system – different organizations and professional groups – must stack up behind one another to achieve the best outcome for patients' (*ibid.*:64).

Over to you

Drawing on the work of Eraut (2003), Hean *et al.* (2008) argue that 'Theory for theory's sake is futile but practice that is not underpinned by a sound theoretical underpinning is tantamount to incompetence'. We have explored the practice scenarios in Part I through the lens of the theories in Part II. We hope that this will provide you, the reader, with new insights, ideas and enthusiasm for collaborative working in its widest sense, not only with other practitioners in health and social care but with service users, carers, wider services, communities and policy makers. As you reach the end of this chapter don't put the book back on your bookshelf but return to the questions at the end of the chapters in Part I to see how your understanding of the issues has developed. As you do this also identify what you think the chapter authors may have missed in their interpretations of the material and what alternative paradigms can be applied. As editors our passion for collaborative working with the outcome of providing a better service for all has sustained us through the writing process. We have recognized how our ideas have developed and, despite the inevitable limitations of this publication, value the knowledge we have constructed as an interprofessional team. We now invite you to take the ideas in this book forward in your own communities of practice and working environments.

References

Barrett G, Keeping C (2005) The Processes Required for Effective Interprofessional Working. In: Barrett G, Sellman D, Thomas J (eds) *Interprofessional Working in Health and Social Care: Professional Perspectives – An Introductory Text.* Basingstoke:Palgrave Macmillan,18–31.

Belbin R (1981) *Management Teams: Why they Succeed or Fail.* London:Heinemann.

Beresford P, Banfield F (2006) Developing inclusive partnerships: user-defined outcomes, networking and knowledge – a case study. *Health & Social Care in the Community* 14(5):436–44.

Bokhour B (2006) Communication in interdisciplinary team meetings: what are we talking about? *Journal of Interprofessional Care* 20(4):349–63.

CAIPE (1997) *Interprofessional Education: A Definition.* London:CAIPE.

Clark P (2006) What would a theory of interprofessional education look like? Some suggestions for developing a theoretical framework for teamwork training. *Journal of Interprofessional Care* 20(6):577–89.

Clarke B, Miers ME, Pollard KC, Thomas J (2007) Complexities of learning together: students' experiences of face-to-face interprofessional groups. *Learning in Health and Social Care* 6(4):202–12.

Crawford M, Rutter D, Thelwall S (2003) *User and Carer Involvement in Change Management: Review of the Literature.* www.sdo.lshtm.ac.uk/ (Accessed 18.01.2008).

Day J (2006) *Interprofessional Working: An Essential Guide for Health-and-Social-Care Professionals.* Cheltenham:Nelson Thornes.

DH (2008) *High Quality Care for All: NHS Next Stage Review Final Report.* Chair, Lord Darzi. London:The Stationery Office.

DH (2009) *Working to Put People First: The Strategy for the Adult Social Care Workforce in England.* www.dh.gov.uk/publications (Accessed 284.2009).

Doel M, Carroll C, Chambers E, Cooke J, Hollows A, Laurie L, Maskrey L, Nancarrow S. (June 2007) *Position paper 09: Developing measures for effective service user and carer participation.* London:SCIE. www.scie.org.uk/publications/positionpapers/pp09.pdf (Accessed 20.05.2009).

Engeström Y, Brown K, Christopher LC, Gregory J (1997) Coordination, cooperation and communication in the courts: expansive transitions in legal work. In: Cole M, Engeström Y, Vasquez O (eds) *Mind, Culture and Activity: Seminal Papers from the Laboratory of Comparative Human Condition.* Cambridge:Cambridge University Press, 369–88.

Eraut, M (2003) The many meanings of theory and practice. *Learning in Health and Social Care* 2(2):61–5.

Fauth R, Mahdon M (2007) *Knowledge review 16: Improving social and health care services.* www.scie.org.uk/ (Accessed 1801.2008).

Freeth D, Hammick M, Koppel I, Reeves S, Barr H (2002) *A Critical Review of Evaluations of Interprofessional Education.* London:LTSN–Centre for Health Science and Practices.

Garrett L, Lodge S (2008) *Working together on the front line: How to make multiprofessional teams and partnerships work.* www.rip.org.uk (Accessed 14.03.2009).

Godin P, Davies J, Heyman B, Reynolds L, Simpson A, Floyd M (2007) Opening communicative space: a Habermasian understanding of a user-led participatory research project. *Journal of Forensic Psychiatry and Psychology* 18(4):452–69.

Great Britain (1989) *Children Act.* London:Her Majesty's Stationery Office.

Great Britain (1998) *Human Rights Act.* London:The Stationery Office.

Great Britain (2005) *Mental Capacity Act.* London:The Stationery Office.

Ham C (2009) *Only Connect: Policy Options for Integrating Health and Social Care.* Birmingham:The Nuffield Trust. www.nuffieldtrust.org.uk (Accessed 9.04.2009).

Hammick M, Freeth D, Copperman J, Goodsman D (2009) *Being Interprofessional.* Cambridge:Polity Press.

Hean S, Craddock D, O'Halloran C (2008) *Learning theories and interprofessional education: A user's guide.* Paper presented at Seminar 3: Theoretical Perspectives on Interprofessional Education: Prioritised Theories from Education, ESRC Seminar Series on Evolving Theory in Interprofessional Education, 5 December, University of West of England, Bristol.

Kennedy I (2001) *Learning from Bristol: The Report of the Public Inquiry into Children's Heart Surgery at the Bristol Royal Infirmary 1984–1995.* London:The Stationery Office.

Laming, Lord (2003) *Inquiry into the Death of Victoria Climbié.* London:The Stationery Office.

Laming, Lord (2009) *The Protection of Children in England: A Progress Report.* London:The Stationery Office.

Loxley A (1997) *Collaboration in Health and Welfare: Working with Difference.* London:Jessica Kingsley.

Oakley A (1984) *Taking it Like a Woman.* London:Fontana.

Payne M (2000) *Teamwork in Multiprofessional Care.* Basingstoke:Palgrave Macmillan.

Race P (1993) *Never Mind the Teaching Feel the Learning.* Birmingham:SEDA Paper 80.

Reder P, Duncan S (2003) Understanding communication in child protection networks. *Child Abuse Review* 12(2):82–100.

Richardson S, Asthana S (2006) Inter-agency information sharing in health and social care services: the role of professional culture. *British Journal of Social Work* 36(4):657–69.

Roulstone A, Hudson V, Kearney J, Martin A, with Warren J. (2006) *Position paper 05: Working together: Carer participation in England, Wales and Northern Ireland.* London:SCIE. www.scie.org.uk/publications/positionpapers/pp05.pdf (Accessed 20.05.2009).

TASC Programme Board (2008) *Putting People First: Transforming Adult Social Care.* London:The Stationery Office.

Tennant M (1997) *Psychology and Adult Learning.* London: Routledge.

Thomas J, Spreadbury K (2008) Making the best use of opportunities for supervision, learning and development to promote critical best practice. In: Jones K, Cooper B, Ferguson H (eds) *Best Practice in Social Work: Critical Perspectives.* Basingstoke:Palgrave Macmillan, 251–65.

Tuckman B, Jensen M (1977) Stages of small-group development revisited. *Group and Organisation Studies* 2(4):419.

Warmington P, Daniels H, Edwards A, Brown S, Leadbetter J, Martin D, Middleton D (2004) *Inter-agency Collaboration: A Review of the Literature.* TLRPIII, University of Birmingham and University of Bath.

Wenger E (1998) *Communities of Practice: Learning, Meaning and Identity.* Cambridge: Cambridge University Press.

Index